LONG COVID: THE JOURNEY FOR HELP

J.D. Claunch M.D.

Practical Neuropsychiatry, Inc.

ISBN: 9798395951885

Cover design by: Catherine Minutillo
Edited by: Catherine Claunch
Library of Congress Control Number: 2018675309
Printed in the United States of America

*This book is dedicated to the twelve patients I will
see this week who all have these symptoms and
worry they are the only ones suffering in this way.
Remember you do not have to suffer alone.*

CONTENTS

CHAPTER 1: SOMETHING IS DEFINITELY WRONG

What Is Wrong With Me?

You absolutely know that something is wrong with you. Maybe you were the most organized person at your job, and now you need a secretary to go through the mail. Perhaps you used to juggle 3 kids, a small business, and still have time to put a four course dinner on the table every night. Now, you wake up dreading your busy schedule of one virtual doctor's appointment and deciding what to order from Grubhub. Your fever has been gone for months, and all of the tests your ten doctors ordered have come back normal. You are getting the distinct impression that these doctors, who once looked at you with such sympathy, are starting to get annoyed by you. One after the next, they have told you to get a therapist and a psychiatrist. Your biggest fear is they will stop filling out the disability paperwork because there is no way you could last one hour doing your old job; though your boss assures you they are holding the position open and want their best employee back as soon as you are well. But you are not "well", no one can tell you what is wrong, and no one seems to have any answers about how you can get better or how long you will be like this. You have Long COVID.

I hear this story every day, often multiple times per day. As a neurologist also trained in psychiatry, primary care doctors have begun putting my name on the referral for these patients. These doctors are not sure if I can help, or how I can help, but they cannot explain what is happening to the patient and hope I can. Or at least, they hope my staff can start fielding the phone calls every day so they can take care of patients who are "really sick".

But you *are* really sick. Maybe other people know how to live like this, but you were so strong before. You used to carry the world on your shoulders and now your parents, spouse, and friends need to carry you. You feel you are alone, that no one else has experienced this and that no one in the world could understand. You have read articles about Long COVID, maybe even joined a Facebook group for "long haulers", but that was too depressing. It did not make you feel connected to a community of fellow sufferers. It just terrified you after you read about a few patients who spent 2 years with the same symptoms and never got better. Is that going to be your future?

The Good News?

Long-haul COVID, as many have learned by now, is an increasingly common disorder. With low estimates of around 100 million who have gotten sick with COVID-19, and nearly a million deaths directly related to COVID, the majority of the discussion in medical journals and politics alike has been about "flattening the curve", making sure people wear masks in public, and getting everyone vaccinated. Articles about patients are mostly focused on the worst atrocities and anecdotes of patients dying alone in a sterile ICU bed with no family members allowed in the building. There are a few articles about people "continuing to be sick for months," and others with vague references to Long-haul COVID, but none of them seem to capture the essence of my patients' experiences.

Even though there is a broad consensus both in medicine and in popular culture that "Long-haul COVID" is real and often debilitating, patients and providers alike seem to have a lot of trouble understanding it. Medicine has transitioned away from making diagnoses based on history and exam findings and more towards testing. In diseases like diabetes or thyroid disease, the patient might as well be an Excel sheet with numbers on it. Surely their symptoms matter, but treatment only changes when the numbers change. Doctors are taught which tests to run and what to do when the tests come back abnormal, but many lose their composure and sometimes even their compassion when the "tests all come back fine". They may think it is great news. You have chest pain, but the tests show no heart attack. You are short of breath, but your lungs are working to give you plenty of oxygen based on the pulse ox test. You feel exhausted, but your thyroid and other hormones are in the normal range. The doctor says it is great that all the tests have come back normal, but that is not your experience.

The Patient's Response

What do you, the patient, think when told this "good news"?

"So you're saying nothing is wrong with me?"

"If all the tests are normal, why do I feel so terrible?"

"Are you saying it's all in my head?"

"You must be missing something."

"But I know *something* is wrong with me…"

I see many patients after they have already had these conversations. I have found there are three common responses to it. Each of these responses is normal, and not a sign of a problem with the patient. They are maladaptive responses surely, but they indicate a failure of our system of disparate and fractured medical care.

Response 1: Despondence

These patients walk in my door with a subtle look of terror that continues throughout the discussion and exam. They have seen so many doctors and "gotten nowhere". When I ask them how I can help, they might even respond "You're my last hope," or "I need you to fix me." They feel depressed and they know it, and everyone else knows it, but if another doctor insinuates they need to be treated for depression, that therapy will somehow fix them, they might kill themselves. They dance around it, emphasize muscle weakness rather than fatigue, chest tightness rather than anxiety. They can't answer questions about their mood or what they enjoy, either saying they are fine or just avoiding the answer entirely. I spend half of the visit convincing them I believe they are sick and that they can get better. If they aren't convinced, they may never come see me again, opting to see a different specialist every few months for second, third, or twelfth opinions. At the end of each appointment I have them convinced, able to explain in their own words the nature of their problem, and motivated to do everything I recommend. At the next follow-up, they have done none of the things we discussed. They can't remember for the life of them what in the world I said other than that I seemed to believe them.

Response 2: Anger

These patients may seem calm initially, a cool face just waiting for the inevitable disappointment. They have often No-showed or canceled prior scheduled appointments because they happen to be having worse symptoms the day of the scheduled appointment and they don't believe I can help them anyway. Within a short time, with a little up front empathy, they admit they really hate their primary care physician (PCP). Sure, they first say they have been looking for a new one. Then they hint that they don't feel a good connection with their current PCP. Later the patient might say they feel the other doctor doesn't listen. But when I say I need their PCP to decide if they need certain tests, they lose it and say they really hate their PCP. Their PCP never listens. They only spend 5 minutes with them. The PCP didn't even examine them last visit. They hate their Rheumatologist who says the tests are all normal and their elevated ANA does not mean anything. And they have seen three other neurologists who said implicitly or explicitly there was nothing wrong with them. While they are grateful for my time, they do not really expect that anyone can or will help them.

Response 3: Exhaustion

These patients are so tired. They look tired. They feel tired. And being around them makes everyone else feel a little tired too. They do not feel sad... unless they start thinking about how tired they are. They give short and simple answers. They feel fine

CHAPTER 1: SOMETHING IS DEFINITELY...   7

otherwise, or so they will say. However, when they fill out the form with questions about other symptoms they check yes on every single one. They have gained or lost weight. They sleep 1 hour per night. Every part of their body hurts. They are dizzy. They feel they can't catch their breath. They sit at home and watch TV, but even watching TV is exhausting. They could not imagine reading a book. Their spouse is worried or mad or depressed because they wanted to be a wife or husband and now they are the patient's parent. Sure, they bathe and dress themselves, but if left alone they would probably just lay in bed and have someone bring the delivery food to their bedside table. They tried a few medications, but the side effects were uncomfortable. They read the book on sleep hygiene, but they sleep fine. Now they say they sleep all the time (even though they checked the box and wrote down 1 hour per night). They always go to the doctor's appointments, but if they are honest, they do not actually expect anyone to help them.

Again, these are maladaptive responses to the medical trauma experienced by Long COVID patients, but they are fundamentally normal responses to what these patients have been through. They have lost something. Typically, what they lost was part of how they defined themselves. Maybe it was work, or creativity, or the ability to give quick, witty one line responses to people. It was a big part of their identity and in losing it, they have lost themselves. They are grieving that lost part of themselves and that is natural, but this is made worse by the repeated trauma associated with trying to get help in our current medical system.

Distressed And Dismissed

These patients are worried and want help, and they feel dismissed by most doctors. Some doctors seem compassionate, but unable to help, often insisting that the neurologist or some other specialist is required to fix an obvious problem. Then the specialist is dismissive. Maybe some specialist says they are going to do "all" the tests to get down to the bottom of it, and then they never see that doctor again, just getting a letter or a call from a nurse saying the thousands of dollars in tests are all normal and they can follow up with their PCP. Despite the doctor not having answers or solutions, they know they must see physicians frequently to keep getting support like approved medical leave from work or disability payments, as well as validation from their families that they have a "real" medical condition.

There is no way I can fully describe (and certainly not defend) the problems associated with how our medical system has become dysfunctional. However, it is a very important component of the suffering and the difficulty seeking help that patients with Long COVID experience. Often, people have idealized expectations of the medical system, thinking a doctor out there will know the test that will diagnose their problem and cure them. Others have had enough exposure to modern medical care that they become skeptical from the start, forcing their doctors to prove their intelligence or compassion before they will listen to the advice given. Both typically leave the office disappointed.

In reality, doctors are just as human and just as limited as any other person. Sure, they know the medical textbooks and may be up to date on the literature, but they are still human. They have neuroses, defense mechanisms, and they are just as driven by their own insecurities as anyone else. The most common result of this is that doctors fall into one of two camps when they lack the tools to either diagnose or treat the cause of their patients' suffering. Some doctors latch onto their strengths, diagnosing something like depression (which as it happens, they do not treat) or a completely unrelated condition (which they can treat but does not fix the main problem) and in optimistic hubris they proclaim victory. Others get very uncomfortable and project their insecurities onto the patient, either overtly or seemingly blaming the patient for their failure to improve. These physicians believe they are there to treat real problems like a clot in a blood vessel or an out of range lab test. They call these problems "organic" while other problems like fatigue, pain, or depression are considered less real unless they can find an "organic" cause to blame.

Many of these doctors are quite compassionate at first.

They may not give any hint to these conflicts until the third time they see a patient. This is almost more traumatic. They listen compassionately, express how much they care, do a thorough exam, and maybe order a bunch of tests. Maybe a second encounter seems productive, lots of results (all good) and continued compassion. It is a bit odd they want you to see a therapist and a psychiatrist, but they did ask nicely. You tried, but no one is taking new patients. Since you are not better you call to schedule a follow up.

This time is different. The once compassionate doctor seems less interested. They make a few vague comments about how they have ruled out everything. They ask if you followed their instructions and got a therapist, but when you say you could not find one, they look at you with disappointment. They are indicating it is your fault you are not better because you did not do what they said. For the next two weeks you cannot get it out of your head. You have wasted six months doing tests and spending co-pays just to be dismissed and told it's all in your head. You would scream if you had the energy. You would cry if you had more tears.

Is This All In My Head?

Sometimes my patients ask me out right, "Do you think it's all in my head?" or more aggressively or despondently, "Just don't tell me it's all in my head." I do not know how to answer. I suppose the simple answer is "of course not", for at least the insinuated question of if they are making it up.

But I am a neurologist and a psychiatrist. Sure, their adrenal glands are contributing, possibly their thyroid, probably some cells in their lungs and blood vessels, definitely the cells in their immune system, but they are in my office because of the head part. I like to think that Long COVID is mostly in their head, or at least their nervous system, since they respond pretty well to my treatments, but the only disease that is "all in someone's head" is a primary brain tumor. Every other condition I am aware of includes other body systems. Inflammatory markers rise during depression and mania spells. Lots of patients with panic disorder also have mild heart rhythm problems. Migraine patients have all kinds of changes in the rest of their body. All of the above symptoms and systems, along with many others, are part of the Long COVID syndrome.

In chapters 2-4 I will discuss the current available science regarding "what" is happening in the head and body of the Long COVID patient, but the question "is this all in my head" is not really about their brain. They know their brain is part of the problem. No one imagines forgetfulness and brain fog come from the toes. The question is about a social stigma regarding psychiatric and psychological diagnoses and their treatments.

Now, don't imagine I am going to give broad approval

or defense of the field of psychiatry. It has a very complex history including more than a few crimes against humanity. Just like other fields of medicine, it has been full of racial and gender bias, industry driven corporate nonsense, and other abuses. But the social stigma is not really about all that. It was infectious disease specialists that infected young black men with syphilis, cardiologists who only studied white men to identify symptoms and treatments for cardiac arrest. Our society has forgiven them for these atrocities. The bias against a depression diagnosis is simply because infections and heart disease are considered more "real" than mood disorders and psychotic disorders.

Is This A Neurologic Problem?

It has always amazed me that neurology has maintained respect from the culture, often more respect than other medical disciplines, while psychiatry is often considered little more than pseudoscience. Perhaps it is my personality, a broad education in the liberal arts, or the fact that I trained in both fields that causes me to have a very hard time understanding the fundamental difference between neurology and psychiatry.

Sure, neurology runs more tests, but most of our patients with pain and headache syndromes, movement disorders, or cognitive disorders do not have an abnormal lab test or findings on brain MRIs. Yet, no one truly doubts that migraine, dystonia, or mixed dementias are real. On the contrary, there are blood tests and abnormalities on imaging that correlate with depression symptoms, manic episodes, and schizophrenia. It definitely cannot be the effectiveness or type of treatment offered. The two fields use the same medications for migraine, epilepsy, bipolar disorder, and schizophrenia. Some believe neurology is focused on areas of damage to the brain while psychiatry is focused on how the brain is not functioning, but migraine is very similar to depression in that both are networks in the brain that are not functioning well. I have treated many patients with mania or psychosis due to a damaged area of the brain. I can point to where a particular location in the brain is not working in a delusion, a panic attack, and even apathy.

The only real difference between neurology and psychiatry is how much stigma is attributed to each disorder and to some degree, over time, the personality of the physicians who are drawn to the two fields. For the remainder of this book, I hope you will try to go on a journey with me. We will discuss a world where we see the brain as a single system, not divided into "more real" neurologic problems and "less real" psychiatric problems. It is my hope to abandon those designations entirely and speak to the biology of a person, the psycho-social construct in which that biology lives, and to do so by accepting the perceptions and experiences of the patients I have worked with to better understand that bio-psycho-social system.

Birth Of A Diagnosis

Before doing this, we must accept one other part of medical history. It is the change I believe to be at the source of our greatest failures. It is at the core of medical science, medical training, and medical practice. It is how we define what problems exist in medicine, and therefore drives how we solve those problems. A famous medical historian once said "In some ways disease does not exist until we have agreed that it does - by perceiving, naming, and responding to it." I cannot speak to C.E. Rosenberg's full intention in saying this, but it is particularly relevant to the current problem of Long COVID.

Many people, patients and doctors alike, imagine that medicine is akin to physics. There are objective physical laws the human body must follow, surely, but in many ways the practice of medicine is truly more akin to alchemy than chemistry. We often only have hints and metaphors, patterns and averages, instead of a truly comprehensive understanding of our biology. Even if we imagined we knew all of the parts, how they all interact in a dynamic system is only vaguely understood. Each year, truths that were held as dogma are abandoned to fit new paradigms. These changes are not made through scientific analysis so much as they are made by vote of committees. Some people imagine we are refining a true knowledge and making it more perfect, but any honest appraisal would accept that what we do not know vastly exceeds anything we know about the human body.

The reality is that we are never really talking about "facts" in clinical medicine. At medicine's best, we are working with good metaphors based on large datasets. We know it too, which is why we want to make our decisions based on large clinical trials. Ideally these trials are designed with appropriate controls and blinding both the subjects and the researchers so that even subtle biases and placebo effects cannot mislead us. If medicine was a science akin to physics we would not need this. In physics, simply refining a theory with a few "experiments" to identify flaws is sufficient to predict an outcome. If physics were like medicine, we would have to shoot tens of thousands of rockets into the air every time a new model is made to confirm the theory is accurate. If physics were like medicine, our rockets would fail as easily as our bodies and our best hope would be that the rocket would land in the right place a little more often than would happen by random chance.

This is not meant to be overly critical of Western allopathic medicine (the way M.D.s and D.O.s are trained). It is the best system we have for now. Any honest look at it, though, would accept there is little chance our science will ever become more like physics. The reason for this is obvious. Each new theory in medicine is dependent on those that preceded it. In the field of logic, no conclusion can be more sound (and comprehensive) than the arguments that lead to it. I will give a few illustrations for this but then I promise I will "get to the point".

The Allopathic (Western Medicine) Model

One of the core principles in allopathic medicine is that whatever is wrong with the body (too much or too little of a function), the treatment should be to provide it with the opposite. This comes from the Greek "allos" for opposite and "pathos" to mean suffering (though pathos also includes all other emotions). So if we were to measure your thyroid level and it is low, we give thyroid hormone to replace it. We call it hypothyroidism, and we give levothyroxine, but it is far from that simple. If a patient's thyroid level is measured many times it will fluctuate widely, though less so than many other hormones. There are also very many cases where the thyroid level is misleading and so we measure the hormone that signals the release of thyroid hormone (thyroid stimulating hormone or TSH). Even this is insufficient as the "range of normal" is debated. It is more appropriate to diagnose someone with a slightly high TSH and many symptoms of hypothyroidism than someone with a more elevated TSH and few symptoms. Many patients will focus on the bright red number and the upward arrow that indicates the lab result is out of the normal range, while a good physician understands there are a hundred different body processes we know of that might change the TSH number, and likely a thousand processes we have never considered. If medicine was like physics, a simple algorithm could do the work of the physician. You would not see a doctor, just get your blood drawn. A spreadsheet would determine which supplements you would take, and no one would ever have more problems.

High blood pressure is another important example. The pressure in the blood vessels is even taught as it relates to physics. The heart pump pushes fluid into the artery system, full of tubes that in a healthy person are flexible like rubber. Each beat increases the pressure (the peak is the systolic pressure we measure) and then the blood drains out of the arteries through tinier vessels into the veins, which decreases the pressure (the trough being the diastolic pressure). Seems simple enough, and since we know which medicines reduce the activity of the pump (fewer beats or making each squeeze less aggressive) we should be able to easily predict how much medicine can reduce the pressure by however much. Engineers do this in cities every day, but unlike the plumbing in your city, your entire system of blood vessels is alive and changing constantly. If the pressure gets too low, different branches dilate or spasm to shift the blood here or there. The body wants very constant pressure in the blood vessels of the head so it will spasm the blood vessels in the digestive system, even the kidneys and other vital organs, to shift the blood towards the heart and the brain. When we give one chemical to reduce the heart rate, that chemical also affects all of the blood vessels in various ways, and the body makes a hundred other chemicals in response to amplify or reduce the effect that our medicine has made. Because of this, we have no way of predicting exactly what will happen, so we start with a low dose of a medicine that has been shown to be generally safe, slowly increasing it and monitoring symptoms and pressures with each adjustment.

Now, to why this is relevant. With more complex issues in medicine such as brain functions or the immune system, there are a thousand types of neurons and a thousand types of immune system proteins in a million configurations with a million combinations of interactions. This makes us much more reliant on metaphors and pattern recognition than with more simple issues like thyroid levels or blood pressure. I will speak a little to the current science of Long COVID, but no matter how clear the science seems, we are never seeing the whole system with all of these dynamic interactions together at once, only parts at a time. We may have hints of truth, but these truths are often decided upon after the treatment is shown to work, to justify why it works in retrospect, and leading to many false conclusions along the way. This leads to a constant reinvention of our diagnoses, and our collective memory is very short, often forgetting our prior misunderstandings.

Ever Evolving Medicine

To illustrate this, I will describe the natural evolution of the diagnosis "Multiple Sclerosis". Any neurology textbook will describe how a French neurologist by the name of Charcot discovered the disease. He identified a patient, someone who worked for his family in truth, who had a group of symptoms. You will find that without fail, these physicians would identify clusters of three symptoms that would be called a "triad". For Charcot, he described patients with this new disease as having 1. Nystagmus, 2. Scanning speech, and 3. Ataxia. I will not detail the qualities of these three symptoms, but Charcot identified them as connected, and searched for other patients with the same three symptoms. He may have ignored other symptoms, and included patients who did not have all three. Then, when the patients died, he would inspect their brains and see how they differed from other brains he had inspected. In the case of multiple sclerosis, as you might guess, the patients seemed to have a particular pattern of scars in their brains and thus the diagnosis became "real".

Over the past hundred years, however, the diagnosis has changed a hundred times. No good neurologist would ever identify patients as having multiple sclerosis based on the original "triad" because so many patients were found to have the same scars with very different symptoms. Also, we now know that there are many different disorders that would have that triad of symptoms. However, had Charcot not been curious, innovative, and organized the syndrome may never have been identified. Charcot's observational process to identify a syndrome is the way medical science advances and it truly requires a unique physician.

Phenomenology In Medicine

At its core, this is called being a phenomenologist. In medical school they do not teach this. They teach the current "science", rarely admitting that this science is often determined by retrospectively justifying why our treatments work and why our lab tests are useful. They teach the syndromes we have agreed upon and the "criteria" patients need to meet them. This model of training has some major errors in it. This training biases the physician to only ask the questions necessary to fulfill criteria for the agreed upon disorders, and often to ignore any additional symptoms. A patient may experience this as the physician not listening to them. Then, if a patient does not meet criteria, either with their history, the exam, or the lab tests, the patient does not get a diagnosis and the physician tells them that "everything came back normal". This is experienced by the patient as being told nothing is wrong with them.

The phenomenologist approaches the patient without such biases. If the history, exam, and lab tests match a known diagnosis, the phenomenologist will make it and prescribe the approved treatment. However, additional information will not be rejected. Perhaps they find another pattern in some patients with additional symptoms. Perhaps they pay attention to which of the 3 approved treatments work best with that new symptom cluster vs the others. It is very different from a purely academic researcher in a few respects. Firstly, academic researchers are very rarely generalists, often having patients/subjects narrowed down before meeting them. A Parkinson's researcher will not see everyone who comes to their PCP complaining of tremor. A multiple sclerosis researcher will very rarely see patients until an MRI, lumbar puncture, or another clinician has done the hard work of diagnosis.

The phenomenologist is much more likely to be a general practitioner or at least have a broader specialty, preferring to see many types of patients. Secondly, the patient is always their patient, as opposed to a researcher who sees the patient for only a short time. While the phenomenologist may have interest in what is unknown, they will practice based on the best available science, and recommended treatments will be in line with standards of care. A researcher may not even know the chemical they give you or if what you get is a placebo, and they may only have good data on how the chemical has affected small groups of humans or larger groups of animal subjects. I will illustrate this with chronic pain.

A standard physician may be using an algorithm they found on a medical website. It says that for knee pain without a torn ligament or evidence of rheumatic arthritis on exam, you start with physical therapy. If the patient returns saying the physical therapy did not work, they prescribe over the counter ibuprofen. If that does not work, they may give a higher dose of ibuprofen or go straight to 2nd line therapy like tramadol. If that does not work, they refer to an orthopedist. That orthopedist runs certain tests like an X-ray or an MRI. Then they offer a procedure or more specialized medical treatments like opiate medications. Maybe they send the patient to a second physical therapist. If the patient does not respond to their treatments, they refer to another orthopedist or a pain specialist who will offer a variety of procedures or medications based on their algorithm.

A researcher will recruit patients who have 5/10 pain in their knee, certain lab findings with certain MRI results. They gather these patients who all look exactly the same and perform one experimental procedure (injecting a chemical into a joint for example) and they record in great detail every reported side effect and every patient's response to the treatment, and they publish an article on it.

A phenomenologist works similar to the standard physician, but they notice some patients describe their pain in a unique way. While most describe the pain as constant and aching, some report the pain as stabbing or throbbing and only on some days. They may help the patient investigate what else is happening on those days, realizing that some patients have patterns of eating certain foods the night before or the day of. Knowing that foods affect the immune system, they may work with patients to try eliminating dairy or some other food from their diet. They find that some patients respond really well to removing dairy while others do not, so they keep looking for patterns to help predict which patients might respond to this or other dietary measures. In most cases, they will work the algorithm at the same time, but they are more likely to consider patterns that the algorithm does not account for and adjust their clinical practice as needed. It is also important to the phenomenologist to keep updated in the literature so they understand which patterns may direct them to which interventions.

The Popularity Of Snake Oil

I will warn you there is a fourth type of doctor. They use a lot of fancy terms and may promote themselves as a specialist. Because some patients respond to dietary change, they presume every knee pain patient has a dairy sensitivity (and may even call it an allergy). Perhaps they read that injecting sugar into the knee has some animal data to support it, so they start injecting every knee pain patient with sugar. Maybe they have read some terribly designed article about an animal model where a few arthritic dogs had evidence of Lyme disease, so they believe anyone with knee pain has chronic Lyme (I will discuss Lyme Disease later) and should be given long term antibiotics. Maybe they read an article in a disreputable journal about a new ultrasound treatment for Lyme, designed to kill Lyme bacteria by sending a certain frequency. The study was done on three dogs and there was no long-term follow up, but it seems reasonably safe and they make $100 for each treatment. Now they have a clinic full of chronic Lyme patients who they inject with sugar once a month and do ultrasound treatments once per week along with insisting everyone stop eating any processed foods and take their patented mix of vitamins. This is not a phenomenologist, a researcher, or a standard physician. While they intend well and may help some patients, they are bad doctors because they are neither acting based on standard medical practice nor are they approaching patients with open eyes accepting the limitations of our medical knowledge. These "doctors" will often be kicked out of medical groups and let their board certifications lapse, finding legal loopholes that keep them from being sued by patients for malpractice.

This fourth type of doctor is quite dangerous. I have met many people who even a standard physician will quickly diagnose with a treatable disease like rheumatoid arthritis, but the patient will already be convinced they have a chronic Lyme infection. While the ultrasound may be safe, however ineffective, rejecting standard of care treatments can lead to severe long term disability. A patient may not feel listened to by the standard doc, and they may miss some information, or may not offer as many treatments as are available, but the standard doc is usually following an approved treatment regimen that has been shown to be generally safe and effective for most patients. I would far rather have a standard physician than someone who does not know or care what the standard is. I would even rather someone whose standard of practice is 10 years out of date because at least at some point the community of physicians approved what they are doing.

Can My Doctor Help Me?

Maybe your primary doctor does not know what to do with you, and that is truly what this book is about. Some of this book is written to help the standard physician realize they will not find solutions for you (yet) on UpToDate, but there are likely treatments that can give you substantial relief. This book is designed to honestly accept the limitations of our checklists, admit that they will not give a diagnosis to every patient, and to help everyone realize tools may be available to help patients even when they do not meet criteria for a particular diagnosis where there are FDA approved treatments. This will be based on the literature, but in some cases we have to admit our literature has been insufficient. In those cases we have to consider symptom patterns that haven't yet been or are no longer given names. We must also acknowledge that we make up criteria often arbitrarily, and patients often have a spectrum of symptoms rather than adhering to a textbook.

All is not lost though. Compared to chronic Lyme and other disorders deemed "not real" by many physicians, Long COVID has been a much more acceptable "phenomenon" by clinicians and academics alike. Each week in 2022, there were between 30 and 60 articles related to Long COVID published in peer-reviewed journals, now there are as many as 150 per week. Sadly, the majority of these have one of two main limitations. Some are well designed studies on small groups of patients (muscle biopsies in 10 patients), which makes it difficult to know if the results can be considered applicable to all patients. Others are giant groups of patients (8000 surveys or charts reviewed) where the results just come back with some percentage having some complaint, not addressing causation or treatment. However, if a simple question is asked, the data becomes a lot more relevant.

Long Covid, Chronic Lyme, And Myalgic Encephalomyelitis

Have there been other medical conditions in the past that have similarities to Long COVID? The answer is a resounding yes. While there is a very controversial and confusing smattering of about 1,000 articles on a similar disorder some call chronic Lyme, they are not as helpful. Chronic Lyme was always too controversial for the treatment data to remain unbiased and directive. Much more helpful are the 10,000+ articles published on a syndrome called "Myalgic Encephalomyelitis" (ME). It sounds like a neurologic diagnosis, but many neurologists have never heard of it. However, there is CDC guidance on ME because when criteria have been proposed for it, an analysis showed that at least 1-2 million Americans fulfill those criteria. It was mostly studied by internists and rheumatologists, and also holds the name "chronic fatigue syndrome," which clearly understates the severity of it. It is most well understood to develop after infectious mononucleosis (yep, the kissing disease that knocked you on your butt for 2 months in high school). Because this disorder often begins early in life, it can have a huge impact on the ability to function over a lifetime, making it a significant societal burden.

Myalgic Encephalomyelitis is extraordinarily similar to Long COVID. The same results are found in blood samples with inflammatory markers, muscle biopsies with inflammation and atrophy, and reports of clinical symptoms and their progression over time. The larger our knowledge of Long COVID grows, the more it closely matches the data on Myalgic Encephalomyelitis (Long Mono?). This makes it relatively easy to decide on what treatments to consider for which symptoms.

While it may seem like a leap, much of the medical sciences make this leap all the time. This cardiac disorder is similar to that cardiac disorder. This immune system disorder is similar to that immune system disorder. This helps build hypotheses to test and directs people to medications and treatments to study. And with over 20 years and 10,000 articles published on ME, it is a very good model to have for Long COVID and informs much of what the following chapters will include.

Can I Get Better?

In the next three chapters, I will discuss the most common symptom categories of Long COVID. The hope is it will be accessible to patients and also informative for medical providers at every level. This will be followed by chapters on treatment options for Long COVID's major components with practical advice and solutions, a review of the physical therapies, the psychotherapies, behavioral approaches, and the pharmacotherapies that have been studied. Patients and clinicians alike can go back to it when they feel they have "done everything possible" and develop hopelessness. There is always more hope, and there are always more things to try if one or another approach fails.

My patients who get better do so by abandoning a search for an individual "magic pill", but instead focusing on a holistic approach, using multiple modalities simultaneously, and entering each new endeavor with courage and resilience. When one medication or physical therapy fails, they do not linger there, but ask what is next. And, my hope is that for you, the next step is to read the rest of this book and buy five more copies to give to your friends.

CHAPTER 2: WHERE DID MY ENERGY GO?

You are so tired. So, so, so tired. Why are you so so so tired? Long COVID comes with a kind of hopeless exhaustion. There are so many levels to it. When you wake in the morning, it seems like you need every ounce of energy to just get out of bed and start the day. Why get dressed when the energy you spend getting dressed makes you want to lay back down in bed? You think, maybe coffee will help, but it just makes you jittery without helping you feel any more awake. Maybe it is what you are eating, so you try healthy foods, without success. You try adding in a lot of protein, but that makes you feel bloated. For kicks you try sugary pastries, and then you get a migraine.

And everyone looks at you like you're just being lazy. You begin to hate every one of them. If they knew how this felt they would at least show a little compassion. Work calls again for their weekly discussion trying to find a reason to stop paying your disability, even though you got sick because they did not protect you by giving you protective equipment. Do you have a fever? No. Do you have diarrhea? No. An intractable cough? Nope. Well then can you come in for a shift on Friday? You know that would be impossible, but how do you explain it? Even going online to order delivery for dinner made you feel like you might need a nap again and they want you to come to work?

Fatigue is extremely common and likely the most debilitating symptom of Long COVID, but the word fatigue is completely inadequate at portraying the hole you are in. That is one of the biggest problems with the old term Chronic Fatigue Syndrome (CFS). It is inadequate. You've done everything they told you to do. They tell you to try to sleep better, but you're in bed 20 hours a day. They tell you to get some exercise, but if you do anything more than walk to the bathroom you feel like your muscles will just fall off. You're not even all that sleepy, and when they test your muscles they say you're strong. But you can't do anything. You don't explain the Grubhub fatigue to anyone because they certainly won't understand the drain on your entire system that it takes to decide between the three restaurants you like. Why else get 3 days worth of food, unless you are hoping it might buy you a brief respite from having to decide anything for a while?

Fatigue is such a terrible feeling without any lab test to prove it, and it cannot be seen from outside your own perceptions. But it is just as real as any other post-COVID symptom. The patients that are the most confused by it are the patients who were always energetic before. They could do a 24 hour shift in the ICU, have drinks with friends, take a quick nap, and then be a mom. Now everyone acts like they are lazy. They feel such enormous guilt that their husband is cooking dinner, not sure if they feel worse for their husband or their kids who have to eat that garbage.

If I can achieve anything with this chapter it is to emphasize how real this fatigue is and to give some perspective on the different components so the readers (patient, family, and physician alike) can start to have a little compassion. You heard that right, I want the patient to have more compassion for themselves. In most of my patients, they may express their suffering and the judgment they feel from others, but if they really open up, the most pressure comes from themselves. I've almost considered adapting the AA 12 steps for this particular symptom.

1. I admitted I am powerless over fatigue and that my life has become unmanageable.
2. I came to believe that a power greater than myself could restore me to functionality.

But it falls apart there. You did what the physicians said. You searched for advice online. You're drinking ginseng. But how do you get out of a 10 foot hole without arms or legs? And if anyone else says you might be depressed, you might just stay in bed all day and eat ice cream.

So, what are the elements of this fatigue syndrome and where does it come from? There is no right answer for everyone. It is usually a combination of multiple factors and they must all be considered to really understand why this is so different from other forms of fatigue.

Myopathy

The first and most obvious component of fatigue, though not necessarily the biggest contributor for most people, is a problem with the muscles. The data on this is sparse for COVID specifically, but the components of both the acute illness, the recovery phase, and the chronic phase have many potential effects on the larger muscles in the body. The first potential impact comes from direct invasion of the virus into the muscle. Some studies emphasize this component, but there have not been any good studies to show that the muscle weakness, pain, and fatigability are directly impacted by a viral myositis (direct infection of the muscle). However, it is definitely a possible mechanism. Many different types of muscle fibers have the ACE2 receptor that allows for the virus to get in there and cause havoc. Local and systemic immune cell dysfunction, however, are more likely to cause the symptoms that concern patients. As discussed in other chapters, while we like to think immune cells are very important, it is the chemicals called cytokines that direct those immune cells and they can have independent effects on the muscle tissue.

They have names like Interleukin-6, 1beta, or 8, Interferon gamma, and tumor necrosis factor alpha. They can cause muscle fibers to break down and break apart even without the virus or the white blood cells getting involved. In fact, we used to use some of these chemicals in medicine to treat infections and autoimmune conditions, and muscle fatigue and pain were very common side effects of just individual cytokines. Start adding on more and more and the cytokine storm, as we like to call it, can lead to a thousand effects on the muscle. Some of which we can see on standard testing and some would require complex lab testing not used in clinical medicine.

EMG, a way to look at the electrical activity of muscles, has been shown in many people with ME/CFS to have alterations of myopotentials (electrical signal within the muscle itself), specifically decreased amplitude (size) and duration (shape). A recent study out of Marseille, France found that there was a marked similarity in the changes to myopotentials. This may sound significant, but even though the M-wave is used to study many elements of the nerve and muscle, the actual shape and size of the M-wave is considered irrelevant and differs from muscle to muscle and placement to placement. So these measures are not useful in clinical practice, but in this controlled research study it confirms that the muscles do have electrical abnormalities which match the symptoms of muscle fatigue experienced by the patient.

None of these tests are used clinically because they do not guide management, so it is not considered by most physicians, and consequently it is not taught as important. However, whenever a test shows a clear difference between patients with a disorder and without a disorder (the predictive value of the test), and the mechanism of the chemical (interferons cause muscle fatigue/pain) match the symptom and are confirmed by changes in the electrical activity of the muscle, there should at least be broad agreement that the symptom is real and relevant even if the testing is not useful.

Energy

There are many other important components to muscle fatigue that cannot be ignored. Muscles require a lot of oxygen and patients with Long COVID have many risk factors for reduced oxygen supply to the muscles. There is a direct effect on the blood vessels during the acute infection. In some cases this leads to very small blood clots or blood vessel spasms that can stop the blood from easily flowing to the muscles. Additionally, Long COVID patients often have a small but measurable reduction in lung function which interrupts the exchange of carbon dioxide and oxygen. Poor carbon dioxide clearance from or poor delivery of oxygen to the muscles results in pain and fatigue. Lastly, if the heart is having difficulty pumping blood, the muscles likewise suffer. While most people do not have significant heart damage from COVID, many patients do develop some symptoms of myocarditis either by direct infection of the virus or post-exposure immune system mediated damage.

So, whether it is a reduction of oxygen delivery to or reduced carbon dioxide removal from the muscles, or cytokines reducing the effective metabolism of the muscle, muscle weakness and pain are very common symptoms of both the acute infection and the chronic post-COVID syndrome. It is extremely important to realize there is a lot of misinformation regarding this in the literature. Just as the data surrounding cognitive complaints in Long COVID is full of discussion related to early small groups without "evidence of brain involvement", there will be many articles arguing that muscle involvement in Long COVID is rare. However, a study showing that 10 people with muscle pain do not have evidence of muscle breakdown does not prove that muscle dysfunction is not playing an important role.

One group of physicians in Denmark performed biopsies of muscles in 16 patients complaining of muscle fatigue over a year after the initial COVID infection. Three out of 4 of those patients had evidence of changes to the muscles including muscle fiber atrophy, atypical regeneration, and changes to either the muscle cell structure or energy processes. Continued inflammation was found in 2/3 of patients,

CHAPTER 2: WHERE DID MY ENERGY GO?   37

and in 3/4 there were changes on biopsy showing abnormalities of the blood vessels in the muscles (mostly in the tiniest blood vessels called capillaries). Oddly, they conclude that these are due to infection of the muscle even though they were so far away from the infection they would have healed if it was due to damage caused by the virus itself rather than all the other changes to the immune system and overall metabolism after the fact.

Critical Illness Myopathy

To complicate the issue further, people who are sick in the hospital can often develop muscle and nerve damage called critical illness neuropathy and myopathy. The exact reason for this is not fully understood and it could have similar causes as what we have already discussed, but it is much faster and can be seen on testing within days or weeks of many illnesses, especially ICU cases. While people usually have weakness from being sick and in bed for a while, there seems to be a much more destructive process in some patients and the exact cause is unknown. The immune system may be a big contributor to this critical illness neuropathy/myopathy, but steroids do not seem to help and often cause a similar problem themselves. This is clearly not the main cause of Long COVID muscle fatigue since most patients with Long COVID never required ICU care, but it is definitely compounded in those cases.

So you are weak, and exhausted, and still the doctors keep saying your strength is pretty good. They are even so kind as to explain to you why you are not actually weak, and to say that the testing came back and showed there were no problems with the nerves or muscles, that the spinal cord was intact, and your brain was sending appropriate signals. So case closed, you're not weak. But you are weak. You can't even get off the couch, but when you tell them they say you need more exercise and have been sitting on the couch too much. Maybe they order physical therapy to give you exercises to do, which you of course do religiously to prove to them you aren't just being lazy. Each time you feel like you've run a marathon, but you don't feel you're building any additional stamina or strength, and when you follow up with the doctor they seem confused about what you need.

While these new studies are showing some problems with the muscles in complex laboratory tests or biopsies, the subtle weakness or damage to the muscles is more complex than mild muscle damage or inflammation. More importantly, there are very few tests to show the muscle problems and there are very few muscle specific treatments in Western allopathic medicine. In truth, the muscle "damage" seen in patients is likely one of the smallest contributors compared to the other components of the general fatigue syndrome, but it plays a very important role. Myalgia, a deep aching muscle pain, is very common. If all the other components of the fatigue syndrome make it feel impossible to get off the couch, and you can hardly breathe when you walk down the hall, having your muscles ache makes the graded exercise I recommend seem like torture. That negative feedback, where the treatment causes pain, can lead to a learned helplessness state that is hard to overcome.

Cardiopulmonary Components

One unique component to Long COVID that was not clearly part of the more well studied post-mono syndrome (Myalgic Encephalomyelitis) is the direct effect on the heart and lungs. Much has been said about the percentage of patients receiving the COVID vaccines and cardiomyopathy. So far, the data makes clear that direct infection of the heart muscle and inflammation associated with the immune response to COVID both have a more meaningful and significant impact on the heart compared to the immune response to the vaccine alone. In one study on hospitalized patients, around 1/3 had elevations in a lab value called troponins, a potential sign of heart muscle breakdown or heart strain. Another study used speckle tracking echocardiography to show 79% of patients had mild heart dysfunction during the infection. This test is quite sensitive, but can be abnormal even without clinical signs. Long story short, evidence of heart damage is seen far more often in people with COVID infections than those receiving the vaccines.

Even after infection has cleared, evidence of cardiopulmonary dysfunction may remain. One recent study of 60 patients hospitalized with COVID found that 3 months post recovery the most common symptom (30% of patients having contracted COVID) was fatigue. While the majority of patients had lung and heart function considered within normal range, a measure called the global longitudinal strain was reduced by around 15%. This did not, however, correlate well with subjective fatigue. Another study showed that over 25% of patients had persistent chest discomfort and difficulty breathing 6 months after infection, which did correlate loosely with slow recovery on CT chest scan abnormalities.

Research focused on patients with complete recovery on CT and X-ray scan suggests decreased lung tissue function is still present. A German study investigating lung function in post-COVID patients found that maximal inspiratory pressure and airway occlusion pressure were significantly impaired, though many variables lead to this change in respiratory muscle function. Another group demonstrated that patients with subjective shortness of breath had reduced ability for the lungs to transfer air by a measure using a small amount of carbon monoxide or nitric oxide as well as capillary blood volume (called DLco, DLno, and Vc respectively). Again, while some of these had some correlation with fatigue, the testing was not sensitive or specific enough to be diagnostic and does not guide management beyond verification that in some cases, poor gas exchange in the lungs may be a relevant factor in the Long COVID fatigue syndrome.

Neurotransmitters

But why does it make you tired to even think about moving? Beyond muscle damage, the cognitive component of fatigue is probably the most debilitating. Again, academic approaches to studying cognitive fatigue have told us a lot about potential mechanisms, but very little about diagnosis and treatment in the clinic. With extremely fancy imaging techniques, and questionably inhumane studies in rats, we have learned about how the chemicals in the brain are involved in the cognitive fatigue process. We have long known that the brain recycles the neurotransmitters, disposes of any excess, and makes new neurotransmitters constantly. In short, the end of the wires spit out little packets of chemicals to send a signal to the next neuron in a space called a synapse.

If those chemicals linger too long, there is a pump to bring the neurotransmitter back into the "end bulb" through a process called reuptake. We can use some medications to stop this process, which leaves more of the neurotransmitter in the synapse. These are called "reuptake inhibitors" and many of our antidepressants use this mechanism to increase the availability of neurotransmitters like serotonin, norepinephrine, and dopamine. These are present throughout the brain, but by far the most prevalent excitatory neurotransmitter is called glutamate. All other neurotransmitters are best understood as subtle modulators of the glutamate neuron activity in the brain. Glutamate is vital for learning, attention, and focus. We reduce the activity of one of the receptors (the NMDA receptor) with many drugs like memantine used for dementia and ketamine now being used in depression and pain management.

But wait, if glutamate helps learning, attention, and focus then why would we block it in dementia and depression? The truth is, we have not even begun to understand how glutamate really works in the brain because it is used in every neural network and process. It is the most potent neuron stimulator in the brain, activating at least 30 types of neuron receptors. Blocking it with ketamine causes sedation at high doses, but at lower doses ketamine causes increased brain activity in multiple networks and has been shown to help chronic pain, depression, and certain measures of cognitive function. So they teach that glutamate is the main "activator" of brain cells, but blocking it a small amount causes more brain network activity in some people.

We are discussing this because many of the leading researchers into cognitive fatigue, which is seen in many post-COVID patients, are actively searching for new ways to utilize these chemical pathways in the brain to understand why the brain gets fatigued with more complex cognitive tasks. Glutamate balance is likely a major part of this process. They know that too much glutamate can be harmful to nerves, actually causing brain cells to die if they are exposed to too much of it. Memantine, which is not an exceptionally potent blocker of the NMDA primary glutamate receptor, was originally designed to slow cognitive decline in Alzheimer's by hopefully reducing glutamate toxicity. Unfortunately, while memantine can help some of the symptoms of Alzheimer's and other dementias, the hope that it would protect neurons was found to be untrue. However, brain fog and cognitive fatigue may be the natural mechanism to reduce activity of glutamate producing neurons in a way to preserve brain cells. Unfortunately, we teach people that people's brains are like computers and since computers do not need to slow down until there is a problem, this protective brain fog is considered an error in the system rather than the potential way of protecting brain cells that is now considered more likely than not.

Synapses

But wait, there is more. One of the most complex and important components of cognitive function, often misunderstood by budding neuroscientists, is how the number of connections in the brain actually affect brain function. People wonder at the giant numbers, with 100 billion neurons (and vastly more microglia) and one quadrillion synapses. That's right, quadrillion is a real number related to a real thing that is in your head. It is 1000 trillion, or a million billion. Numbers like these are used to wow the scientific crowd and to describe how powerful the brain's capacity is, as if it is a computer. The more synapses the better, right? Not exactly.

In early life, the rapidly expanding number of synapses may be connected to the development of consciousness, perception, and language as well as creating networks for skills unique to humans. Fewer engrained reflexes (like animals who need a reflex to grab a tree branch to survive as they jump) give way to novel adaptations like the ability to worry about things that do not exist, the human's greatest evolutionary leap forward. As those brain networks begin to solidify, a very important process called "pruning" occurs where the brain starts to remove redundant and unhelpful connections while strengthening the more useful (or at least more frequently used) connections. This pruning process, starting in late adolescence and continuing into the mid-20s, seems to be faulty in people with disorders like schizophrenia, which typically manifest during that period.

Imagine trying to build a city. Roads are necessary and only having a few roads would be terrible for the functioning of a growing population. The more roads you have the better, until things start to get crowded and then you have to make some larger roads with quite regulated onramps and offramps. Imagine if the interstate through your town let every small side street and alleyway make their own onramp? More and more studies are questioning and discovering errors in this synapse production and pruning process associated with "brain fog" and cognitive fatigue.

So now that we have had a small class on brain cells, the chemicals that are involved in increased focus and attention, and some of the proposed mechanisms for cognitive slowing, what can be done about it? Step one is to realize that people spend their entire childhood and young adult life unconsciously creating ways to compensate for the stress the world puts on them. These strategies can be healthy or unhealthy, but since the world keeps spinning, so must we. Let's examine some of the strategies that naturally develop and how they are stripped away by Long COVID.

Routine And Ritual

Day to day routine is vital for people to keep their brains healthy and efficient. While it is impossible to truly correlate the above science on the microscopic components with the lived experience of patients, the themes writ large do match. You wake up at 7am, have cereal, get a shower, get dressed, drive to work where you do a similar job each day, drive home, reflexively order dinner from one of just a few restaurants, watch a show, and go to bed. Most of your decisions are reflexive and habit. Maybe those habits are healthy, maybe they are not, but your pre-COVID brain was very efficient. It really only made a handful of decisions each day. Most of your daily activities were determined by those neural interstate connections, not using any unnecessary glutamate, and physically tiring yourself out by the end of the day (which ends after a specific evening routine) so your brain knows it is bedtime.

But then you got sick, and the world you knew collapsed in on itself. You wake up and have to decide what is next. Your brain is spinning with fear about how long your sick leave will last, what you can do without 3 days of feeling like you got hit by a bus, and if you should try to find more restaurants with their own delivery service because you heard those national food delivery services are a scam. Because each day is different, and also exactly the same, they blend together. You have to work to remember about 5 times that you already took your morning medications. You have to decide each day if you should pay attention to what day it is. You've worried about so many things, and made so many individual decisions, that your brain is filled to the brim with glutamate use by around 10 am, and you don't know why it feels like bedtime already.

Over the past few months, your synapses have lost the ability to know what connections are important and routine, and which are extra and unhelpful. Your brain is building onramps from each little side street and a year of twilight sleep instead of deep restorative sleep has overwhelmed the glymphatic system so the sewage is backing up, slowing down traffic even further. So you lay on the couch, staring at the ceiling, deciding if you should go to the bathroom now and if it will be worth the leg pain it will cause. Your brain takes about 10 minutes to decide it just is not worth it yet. Now, imagine that only a very small part of your brain processing is even in conscious awareness. Since you don't walk every day, your brain is struggling to figure out which brain connections to strengthen or prune for balance, coordination, keep track of time, engage with other people, and of course consider every possible catastrophe if this lasts much longer.

So your muscles are tired, surely, and they ache. But the fatigue your brain is experiencing is likely more important. While it is kind of depressing to realize how much of your activities and thoughts were on autopilot, when that autopilot is gone and there are suddenly infinite more decisions you have to make each day (consciously and especially subconsciously), exhaustion is to be expected.

Fatigue And Depression

While I find the psychological underpinnings to all of this fascinating and vitally important in treating patients, it is also laden with stigma. It could be viewed simply as behavioral conditioning, with pain on every step leading to learned helplessness and inactivity. There are evolutionary psychology models that would insist that physical inability leads to depression and inactivity in order to reduce pulling resources from the group. There are obviously many overlaps between the neurochemical development of fatigue and the same networks and symptoms involved in depression. However, the moment the word depression is used, our society imposes stigma and misunderstanding. Maybe you have childhood memories of depressed individuals being called lazy or weak. Maybe you have been depressed in the past but this is different. Maybe last time you got better with the power of positive thinking, and this seems more like a "real medical problem".

Well, it will be hard to avoid discussing depression in the Long COVID syndrome since it is pervasive. Do we avoid using the term or does that further stigmatize it? Do we just talk of depression in terms of brain networks and ignore the social, spiritual, and existential underpinnings? This is an extraordinarily difficult topic because when a word has a thousand meanings, it ceases to have any meaning at all. As time has progressed, the term depression in the field of medicine has become a categorical syndrome designed to make it easy to study.

Depression has been distilled down to just a few symptoms: 1. sadness, 2. inability to feel pleasure, 3. changes to sleep and appetite, 4. low energy, and 5. thoughts of suicide or self harm. It is still allowed to have melancholic or psychotic features, but what of dread, emptiness, and angst? Have the other thousand human experiences lost meaning because they have not made their way into the medical model of depression research? What many do not know is that research at the National Institute of Mental Health has also been shifting funds to divorce itself from the classic psychiatric syndromes (major depression, generalized anxiety disorder, panic disorder, schizophrenia) and move towards equally arbitrary ideas like Acute threat (previously known as Fear) and Potential threat (previously known as Anxiety) as well as Frustrative non-reward, a concept created by researchers to describe their journey through academia.

To the academics, these seem like measurable terms with distinct neural mechanisms. They hope these terms overtake the diagnosis of depression in research, and eventually management. They hope that better drug choices can be made with more accurate symptom clusters. This has done nothing to improve patient care, yet has reduced funding for studies investigating the classic syndromes (however imperfect they are) still used by nearly all providers, and has made the literature more disjointed.

However complex and disjointed the field has become, the current model for treating depression and anxiety has been shown to be as or more effective than treatment of nearly all other medical conditions. This does not mean it is easy, and it does not mean patients have access to this treatment. Medications are vital, but they are not enough. Treatment of the mood component, which manifests as depression, apathy, low energy, anxiety, panic, and/or hypervigilance, involves close monitoring, medications that affect serotonin, norepinephrine, and dopamine in the brain as well as various forms of therapy including behavioral activation, CBT for sleep, stress reduction therapies, mindfulness, cognitive reframing, and a whole host of acronyms like DBT, EMDR, ACT, and IFS. All have a major role in treating the symptoms of depression, and with treatment of the depression syndrome comes improved physical and cognitive functioning.

The Key Is In The Box

Unfortunately, my patients consistently tell me they have been too exhausted to do therapy, exercise, cook healthy foods, and meditate. The old psychology analogy for depression truly fits with Long COVID fatigue. If you could just open the box, then you would have the key needed to open the box. Your doctor's advice sounds simple when they say it, but they just do not seem to understand how difficult it is to do it. The problem here is that this requires a lot of help and strategizing. It requires a very individualized approach, since the barriers to changing behavior are always unique to any patient. Even strategizing seems to use up an enormous amount of energy. This is often where therapy can be extraordinarily helpful. The problem is that even finding a therapist (physical therapy or psychotherapy) is extraordinarily hard these days. Patients have a real and reasonable fear that they are going to wait on a waitlist for two months, spend another 2 months telling their life story, and this precious time and energy will have been wasted if they didn't pick the right therapist.

I find a few key principles can speed this process along. Step one should be trying to identify an advocate helper. This could be a family member, a friend, or a case manager. They can help you organize your search, advocate for a sooner appointment, and keep you honest in your search so you stay motivated to keep trying rather than give up (however rational giving up may seem). Step two is to put your eggs in multiple baskets. Get on 3 wait lists instead of 1. Try to identify a physical therapist, an acupuncturist, and a talk therapist so you are not trying to fully rely on just one modality to help. Step three should be to understand what type of incentives you respond to best. Do you like to have someone push you harder or slowly encourage you? Do you do well with homework or do you need more frequent sessions to stay motivated? With no judgment on this, recognize what has worked to motivate you in the past and admit that to the therapist you meet. Step four is to give any therapist an honest try, at least 3-4 sessions, making sure to let them use their method, but honestly saying when you are not sure where things are going. Step five is to terminate with the therapist in a session (after you have given them 3-4 sessions) by talking about why you think things are not working. This can either lead to a new arrangement with new methods or a referral to someone else who might match your goals and motivations better.

Lastly, stay as hopeful as possible until you quit. Worrying, pessimistic thinking, and hopelessness are perfectly rational at times, and the goal should never be to rationalize them away. You accept that worrying is rational, and at the same time practice focusing on hope as fully as you can (for a set and very limited amount of time) even if it is irrational. Trying to live hopeful forever can be harmful and lead to waste, but if you do not believe something will help it is far less likely to. This is one of the hardest things for patients to practice and physicians are very unskilled at helping it along. They may say everything is going to go well if you do therapy, ignoring the rational fears you bring and thus not addressing them. Alternatively, they may amplify the fear, saying that therapy may not help but if you do not do therapy you will get even worse. If they do this, just realize that this sort of complex motivational skill is not taught in medical training, and you should work on this with your advocate and then with your therapist, who will likely be better.

But never let anyone begin to convince you to believe the fear, the fatigue, the pain, and the hopelessness are irrational, your fault, or "all in your head". These emotions, thoughts, and experiences are not always helpful, and with the skills in your head and body you can temper them, but they are quite real and not your fault. This thing happened to you, it was real, and it is traumatizing. This should not be denied, but it is only the beginning of the story. People do get better. People get better in unpredictable and surprising ways sometimes. Sometimes people are the last to know they are getting better because it takes a while of being better to feel better. And while it is hard to obtain, help is out there in many different disciplines from pulmonologists looking for sleep apnea, to psychiatrists prescribing depression and attention medications, to physical therapists helping with an exercise plan. Without hope, it is much harder to make the phone call, schedule the appointment, and keep up with the exercises. The best part is that after hope, medications and exercise become the habit, the ritual, and the routine. They can naturally reduce fear, fatigue, and hopelessness. Problem solved, right? Stay hopeful, do the work, and the fatigue can improve. But now you're thinking, "what did I just read? Did I agree with what he just said?" In the next chapter, we will discuss why you will need to re-read this chapter a few times since you cannot remember anything anymore.

CHAPTER 3: WHY DOESN'T MY BRAIN WORK?

Cognitive symptoms in Long COVID can persist for months or more after acute infection. However, they are also the most difficult for patients and providers to talk about. It is as if there are three separate languages, using very similar terminology, but with each term having completely different associations and meanings. Neurologists, neuropsychiatrists, and patients all use the same words when speaking about cognitive functioning, but they all mean very different things by those words.

Memory is a great example. I see a dozen new patients each week who say their main problem is their memory, but after a full assessment, memory is not my concern. They disagree and go on to give me twenty very clear and detailed examples in the past two days of things they forgot. It does not help them feel any better when I tell them it is a good sign they remember they forgot. It's all the more frustrating when they can remember that every person in their family has told them their memory is terrible, and their primary care doctor agreed at their appointment. Why does the neuropsychiatrist disagree?

Memory

Memory is not just one thing, and people (including many physicians) rely more on a colloquial definition of memory than what we look for on our neurological exams. Even the screening exams (the Montreal Cognitive Assessment and the Folstein Mini Mental Status Exam being the most common) are very poor tests to measure the actual individual brain functions that we call memory. They are, at best, a good measure of the combined activity of attention and memory. It seems like it should be simple enough. Forgetfulness is a pretty good term to use, but is not always accurate. For someone to genuinely forget something, they must have learned it in the first place, and then have difficulty retrieving it. If I have an appointment at 2pm and I "forget about it," then someone asks me what I have going on that day and I immediately respond, "Oh, crap! I forgot about my appointment!" then I didn't actually forget about it. I put it back into a file and then got distracted by something else, and my real problem is easy distractibility (or poor attention).

The cognitive complaints associated with Long COVID are extraordinarily diverse both in nature and cause, memory being just one concern. We should, however, discuss memory at some length so the nature of cognitive complaints can be understood in their complexity. We will start with the example of how sounds (like someone telling you something) become memories. It begins with hearing. The sound waves have to get turned into perceived sound and filter through the attentional networks in the brain that say "pay attention to this". There are about 20 steps to that process even before the language networks get involved. The first steps include a quick analysis of who is saying it, how they are saying it, and key parts of the sounds as well as mechanisms to separate those sounds from background noise. Depending on how these subconscious processes occur, hearing a noise may not result in registering the noise as someone telling you something (or registering the noise at all). These mechanisms are why after 40, people often have difficulty following a conversation in a crowded room (called presbycusis) and men often do not "hear" the women they should be listening to.

It is only after the sound is flagged as important and distinct that the brain turns those sounds into concepts. This requires the language networks throughout the entire left hemisphere of the brain. This process is modulated by the right hemisphere to account for tone, affect, and even cadence to give context. The right hemisphere helps decide if "she is on fire" means she is good at something, very attractive, or in the middle of an emergency.

Once the information is deciphered using these interconnected networks, the brain (once again) decides if it is important information. If all the processes occur properly, the information finally enters "working memory", which is not memory at all. Working memory is another type of attention where this information finally enters "awareness". Only after it cycles around the Papez circuit a few times is it re-encoded, manipulated, paired with other flags and contexts associated with other memories, and finally stored in bits and pieces in various areas of the brain.

Finally, after all that, as a neuropsychiatrist, I can comfortably call it a memory (something experienced, then learned, and then stored). Then comes the hard part, where you have to get that information back out of storage when you want it, how you want it, and with some level of accuracy. Obviously we do not continually access all of those memories, so there has to be a trigger to tell our brain we need that information.

The trigger could be cues (like the doctor asking what those 5 words were he asked you to remember) or the activation of other memories it is paired with. This is how people "train their memory," by practicing associations called mnemonics. I want to remember my dental appointment, so my brain connects it with the date and other tasks for the day. I remember that it is Tuesday, which comes after Monday (negative emotional valence), and I get to leave work early (positive emotional valence) because I have a dentist appointment (negative emotional valence) I will probably remember it. If I want to give myself a better chance of remembering, I'll also realize that Tuesday kind of sounds like Tooth Day and my brain, loving puns, will repeat that joke to a few people further solidifying the connection.

However, when I get home I realize I forgot something. Something serious. What was it? Oh crap, I forgot to get milk on the way home, even though I now remember in great detail that my wife told me to get her milk on my way out of the door this morning. But having "forgotten" it does not have anything to do with my memory. It was because I had 4 other things stealing my attention (more in another book on how attention is actually directive inattention) because they had stronger emotional pull to keep them back on my mental television screen rather than the storage cabinet where the memory of my wife's needs were left (forgotten in my memory if you will).

So why did I go down this tangent? I won't blame you if you've forgotten. I know I almost did. I am talking about the complexity of memory in the brain because deciphering why post-COVID patients have difficulty with remembering things is far more complex than it might initially seem. However, due to pretty modern scientific research, we understand a lot about what is happening to the brain during and after COVID as well as how it relates to a lot of these complex cognitive functions.

Brain Networks

Are you ready for some overly simplistic neuroscience? At the very center of the scientific debate around cognitive complaints in the setting of COVID are a group of brain cells we have always neglected to talk much about. Early in the field of neuroscience, we became obsessed with the neuron. Neurons are the cells that we typically talk about the most because they act like little computer processors. They connect to each other and stimulate each other. When a big cell body gets enough stimulation from other neurons, it sends a small bio-electrical current down an axon, which functions like an electrical cable, sending "information" to other neurons, and so on and so forth. Memory is when these neurons link together in certain ways to make connections stronger and stronger. So, when I think of August and remember my wife's birthday, the neuron(s) responsible for the 'August memory' and the 'wife memory' form stronger and stronger connections until the memory is more and more ingrained, hopefully preventing me from forgetting to get her a gift. All of this is at the core of our understanding of the brain, taught in every first year neurology and general psychology course, and it is all fundamentally a lie. I suppose all things we teach and learn are just metaphors, but it is both a lie and a terrible metaphor.

The truth is, while we know neuronal connections and activity play a big role in brain functioning, how connections form into memories, thoughts, feelings, actions, etc. is extraordinarily complex. It also involves many other types of cells that are vital in establishing those neuronal connections. Glial cells nourish these connections, protect them, and then remove them as needed. In fact, this last process, called pruning (yes, like in gardening) is possibly the most important task because too many inappropriate connections can lead to as many problems as not enough.

Trying to help people envision this is very difficult. There are many diagrams out there, but none do it justice. Suffice to say that if I see a hundred patients for "memory complaints", maybe one in that hundred have a primary neuron degeneration problem. It is far more likely I identify a neuron degeneration problem in a patient with changes to their coordination, a tremor, or a tic disorder than in someone with memory problems. On the rare occasion I meet someone with a neuron problem leading to memory troubles, the patients are typically completely unaware of it. These are Alzheimer's patients who think they are just fine even though they cannot tell me who their daughter is that brought them. The vast majority of people complaining of cognitive slowing, and nearly everyone with Long COVID brain fog, have problems with the connections in the brain. Their networks are misbehaving because of the glial cells, not the neurons.

Other Brain Cells

Glia (meaning glue from the original Greek) is a generic term for three main categories of cells that all play a vital role in brain structure and functioning. The glial cell most people first think of is the oligodendrocyte (Greek: cell with a few branches), which sends projections to wrap and protect the axons (like insulation around an electrical cable) throughout the brain. These are the cells damaged in many brain inflammatory conditions such as MS. Generally, investigations have shown oligodendrocytes to be spared in patients with post-infectious conditions like Long COVID. One recent study, however, suggests there may be some changes to the production of new oligodendrocytes in the hippocampus, which plays a role in the working memory circuit we described. Rarely, an infection can activate a previous autoimmune condition that directly attacks these cells. During or after COVID, however, we have not seen obvious cases of direct damage or dysfunction to most of the oligodendrocytes in the brain.

The second type of glial cell that plays an extraordinarily important role in brain health is the astrocyte, named such because they look like little stars. They are the worker bees of the brain, performing dozens of tasks. Of vital importance, they are responsible for forming the blood-brain-barrier (BBB) along with another special cell called a pericyte (Greek: the "cell next to" the blood vessel). The BBB has the critical task of keeping toxins and other chemicals in the bloodstream from entering the brain. Astrocytes form this barrier by wrapping around the tiniest blood vessels called capillaries. They also supply neurons with energy, regulate metabolism, and likely are responsible for telling neurons where and how to wire with other neurons. Astrocytes also share receptor types with neurons, and may even play a role in signal creation, activating and deactivating neurons. Of all the brain cell types studied, astrocytes may be the only ones where there is good evidence of direct infection by a variety of these viruses that have post-infectious syndromes, including COVID. There is not, however, good evidence to show that direct infection of astrocytes is related to symptoms such as brain fog.

Microglia are the third main category of glial cell and they may be the most consistently altered cell type in syndromes like Long COVID. The astrocytes and their BBB keep the rest of the immune system separate from the brain, but the brain has its own immune system in the form of microglia. When inactive, they are pretty dormant, working as general support cells for the astrocytes. However, whether due to illness, injury, or some other process, they can be activated, which makes them swell up and change their function entirely. Just like immune cells in the rest of the body, how they are activated can give them many goals. They can attack infections, clean up waste from damaged brain cells, and cause a lot of havoc along the way. While there is not yet data of direct infection of microglia by the COVID virus, patients with prolonged symptoms after COVID almost universally have activated microglia throughout their brains. If there are 1,000 activated microglia under a microscope, they are doing 10,000 separate tasks, so investigating all of the consequences of this is impossible.

Lastly, as mentioned before, blood vessel changes can be seen throughout the body after a COVID infection, and the brain is no different. The endothelium (the innermost lining of the blood vessel walls) is both prone to infection and dysfunction during and after COVID infection. It is not enough to allow blood to get through, but it definitely leads to changes in what is allowed into the brain and what is kept out. Along with dysfunctional astrocytes, damage to the capillaries can lead to less energy entering the brain, and difficulty keeping toxins in the bloodstream out of the brain.

All of these problems, from activated microglia to disruptions in the blood brain barrier have very significant, but difficult to study, effects on the way the brain functions. These changes are not detected by standard screening measures such as CT scans, MRIs, and blood tests. Even lumbar puncture, which looks at the fluid on the other side of the blood brain barrier, the cerebrospinal fluid (CSF), is unreliable. We rarely see significant changes on standard CSF testing until enough damage occurs that brain cells start dying. However, when we look for proteins associated with immune system function in the CSF, there is a significant elevation in many cytokines including CCL5/RANTES, IL-2, IL-4, CCL3, IL-6, IL-10, IFN-γ, and VEGF. These proteins may be responsible for activation of the microglia by leaking through the damaged BBB, but cause and effect are unclear. Glial cells may create these cytokines in response to other proteins entering through the BBB. One thing is clear though, all of these changes are present in patients with Long COVID symptoms, and not in healthy folks who did not develop symptoms after infection.

Glymphatics

There is another function of the glia that is poorly understood but considered essential for overall brain health. The glymphatic system helps the brain clear toxins, especially while people sleep. It is impossible to study in relation to individual disease processes, but problems with the glymphatics can play a role in almost all brain disorders. The glymphatic system is created and controlled by the glia, so disorders where the glia are disrupted or activated are presumed to reduce the effectiveness of this drainage process. It is not helpful to think of this as a cause of the acute process of COVID confusion or even the post-acute sequelae, but disruptions in glymphatic flow likely play a role in the slowing of recovery for many patients.

Cortical Symptoms

It is not surprising that patients never come to me worried about their glymphatic system. Universally, they tell me they worry about dementia, specifically Alzheimer's. Poorly written news articles about "Alzheimer's changes" after COVID infection have some patients particularly alarmed. This is especially true for anyone who has watched a family member decline with a diagnosis of Alzheimer's disease. One of the first things I tell them, which does not always help, is that the more worried a patient is about Alzheimer's, the less likely they are to have it. Genuine Alzheimer's disease, like many other scary dementias, is a degeneration of the cortex of the brain (the outside layer where most neurons live). One of the first symptoms is loss of insight, which means they are not aware of a problem. In short, it is a good sign patients remember they forgot, they are worried about it, and they are seeking help.

Until recently, the diagnostic criteria for Alzheimer's disease included language specifically related to the three main "cortical symptoms" that have been understood for a century. They are the apraxias, aphasias, and the agnosias. Praxis means task, and A-

Praxia means loss of the ability to do certain tasks. Like Ariel from *The Little Mermaid* combing her hair with a fork, people with praxis difficulties lose the ability to use simple tools correctly. This is different from difficulty learning new tools like a different type of cell phone, but it can be difficult to differentiate from generalized confusion in its early stage. A-Phasia means loss of a language function (I won't get into how aphasia is not the right word from the Greek since it should be dysglossia, but that word was taken). Many patients with good neurons will have mild word finding trouble or stuttering, but people with aphasia have sometimes very subtle changes that only pop up when you pay close attention. They sometimes lose the ability to use or understand complex syntax. "The Lion was eaten by the Tiger" is indistinguishable from the "Lion ate the Tiger". If a sentence has more than one comma, they do not just lose attention half way through (like you may have while reading this book), they truly cannot understand what is happening. They may also use a lot of incorrect words, called "paraphasias". Instead of "I ate a banana", they say "I ate a bonobo" or "I ate a bana". Lastly, gnosis is "to know" and A-Gnosia means to lose awareness of something. Lack of insight or denial of illness is a great example.

This can be pretty difficult to understand unless you see a lot of people with genuine pure Alzheimer's as well as a lot of people with other causes of forgetfulness. Where a drowsy, inattentive person may forget to put the right detergent in the washer, a person with apraxia will put detergent on the clothes and put them first in the drier, or start washing their clothes in the dishwasher. They may put their underwear on the outside of the pants or start trying to write a letter with a knife instead of a pen. A good general rule is, when people feel like a task takes 10 times as long, it is a subcortical (read attention/concentration) problem, but when they ruin their clothes or the clothes drier, they might have a cortical problem.

Alzheimer's patients are almost always brought in by family members. The big tip-off to diagnosis is how the family member acts and talks. When discussing any other topic they may use very short sentences (so the patient can understand), but when they talk about the memory problem, they start using very complex sentence structure. Below is a typical encounter.

Neurologist: "How is Mom's mood?"
Daughter: "She's doing great."
Neurologist: "How is Mom enjoying living with you now?"
Daughter: "She's glad she's here."
Neurologist: "What makes you think there is a memory problem?"
Daughter: "I'm particularly disquieted, and so is the primary care doctor, that Mom might be slowly developing concerning signs of a degenerative condition."

The patient's daughter is not even aware she is making her language more complex, but these adaptations slowly develop to avoid conflict. The patient does not pause to gather her thoughts, but speaks with normal speed. She uses the wrong words or strange phrases in very short sentences. This is very different from the concussion patient or the sleep apnea patient who very slowly tells me their story with starts, stops, and stuttering.

Gnosis errors are probably the most obvious. When I ask a patient what they did this morning, she will say she went out for breakfast, but her daughter is shaking her head because it isn't true. It is not forgetfulness, or a slow partial answer, but a quick false response that points towards cortical brain damage. It is called confabulation, and the response is often quicker than a healthy person. The human brain is constantly making up things, like imagination, but very specific areas (in the right frontal lobe) are designed to double check before responding. With this area's reduced activity, the other areas are capable of running amok and giving false answers. Gnosis errors are not forgetting someone's name, they are confusing their daughter for their mother or thinking the fork is a pen.

Now, I do not mean to say that all cortical problems are Alzheimer's dementia, but if you have severe deficits and none of them are cortical, then it probably is not Alzheimer's. Other common causes of cortical deficits are chronic alcoholism (which often has both cortical and subcortical deficits) and active delirium. Delirium is when someone has a fragile brain and they get a medical illness. Both of these conditions can have cortical deficits, but they also have subcortical deficits. It can be argued that some psychiatric disorders such as psychosis can involve prominent cortical dysfunction.

Subcortical Symptoms

So what are subcortical deficits? In short, they are problems with the connections in the brain. Beneath the cortex (where most of the neurons live) is the white matter, where the wires are that connect neurons in one area of the brain to neurons in other areas. These axons are affected by many different medical conditions including inflammation, small strokes, and weakening of the capillaries in the brain. The list of medical conditions that cause a weakening of these connections is endless, and the resulting symptoms can be either permanent or can resolve when the contributor is treated. For one person, it is diabetes and insomnia. Another person will have subcortical dysfunction from depression and hypertension. A theory called allostatic load has been proposed as the reason for this. Any one disorder (or exposure) would not cause problems with memory or other brain functions, but as they add up they can compound on each other.

So what are these symptoms? Honestly, it can be anything besides the primary cortical deficits. Slowed difficult thinking, easily doing a simple task but missing steps with more complex tasks, taking a long time to remember a name or a word, or the dreaded failure of your autopilot. Sometimes autopilot failure makes you drive to work instead of going to pick up your child from school. Sometimes it takes you to the bathroom, initiated by a thought you had 5 minutes ago, and you think to yourself "Why am I here?" Subcortical deficits can lead to significant difficulty forming memories. You cannot consistently get memories from your attention to the storage areas or you have difficulty getting memories from storage into working memory again. In this way, forgetfulness is just as likely to be subcortical, but you typically have insight about having forgotten or having difficulty recalling.

Brain Fog

In COVID, there can be a variety of different symptoms depending on other contributors. During the acute illness, patients can have delirium causing a combination of cortical and subcortical deficits. This can also be true if patients have other active medical issues, or if insomnia is present. After "the dust settles" and the COVID infection has resolved, the deficits are almost universally subcortical. Patients describe it in so many ways. They are walking through life dazed, off, in a fog, groggy, or as if their battery has been removed. They cannot speak a full sentence without getting lost on the way. Some patients feel hungover, or even a little drunk. Others say they feel like they took benadryl or a bunch of cough medicine. Some worry they are still sick since they felt similarly when they had a cold or flu in the past.

Mostly, they feel lost. They were always sharp and funny, but now they can hardly think straight. They can't tell if an hour or half the day has passed, and each day runs into the next. Maybe they eat all day, or maybe they just forget to eat, especially since food still tastes like chalk ever since they lost their sense of smell. They have low energy, can't enjoy anything, feel tired but can't sleep or sleep all day, and they can't concentrate. They try to read a book, but find they can't remember what the beginning of the paragraph said when they get to the end. So they try to listen to an audio book, and they realize they can't follow it, or maybe they fell asleep for a while and didn't notice.

They don't feel depressed, but they have all the symptoms of depression. Patients say their body or their brain is depressed, not them. Fundamentally, the same thing is happening to their brain as what happens during an episode of depression: reduced energy and functional connectivity of the frontal lobes and the limbic system of the brain. All the areas of the brain involved in pleasure, motivation, energy, focus, interest, and attention have reduced activity, but so far, as in depression, there is no evidence of damage to those neurons.

Brain Scans

While imaging designed to show structural problems in the brain (MRI, CT) is typically unhelpful in post-COVID patients, some types of imaging do show changes. FDG-PET scan is a very fancy way of looking at the overall and regional function of the brain. In this specialized scan, we give patients special sugar marked to show up on the scan. Areas light up to help us determine what areas of the brain or other tissues are using energy and how much. For example, if you scanned a person's muscle at rest and then scanned them during or right after exercise, the muscle would show a significant increase in signal on the FDG-PET scan. Comparing two different people would be like comparing apples and oranges since metabolism is such a unique process from person to person and moment to moment. This scan is only really useful to compare areas of muscle or areas of brain tissue.

FDG-PET scan has limited usefulness clinically, but research studies have shown a connection between easy muscle fatigue, cognitive slowing, and energy use within the muscles and brain. From this research we can at least say "something is going on." A group out of France led by Drs. Gudej and Eldin, as well as other groups, have found consistent changes specific to certain areas of the brain in Long Covid patients with cognitive slowing. The frontal lobes (involved in behavior), the right side of the brain in the limbic areas (memory, emotion, and behavior regulation), and the thalamus (kind of the regulator in charge of activating and deactivating those other areas) all appear to be affected. In some people, there was also reduced activity in the pons (deep brain stem). In addition to other roles, the pons is an activating center for the whole brain, regulating alertness.

Unfortunately, the FDG-PET is not a very specific test since it does not just look at neurons. Changes in metabolism (measured by FDG-PET) can be seen if the support cells of the brain are not as active or overactive. Also, if one cell type is overactive and one is underactive it may show no changes on the scan at all. Lastly, even if neurons are overactive, that might be a compensation measure because the activity of those cells is not as effective or streamlined as it should be. This makes a clear interpretation of the results of these studies difficult, but there is no question that there are changes to the brain's functioning in these patients. Fundamentally, while imaging and lab work are helpful in research to determine patterns and investigate treatments, they are not helpful in diagnosis or determining which would be the most useful treatment in most cases. If they are used, it is mainly to determine if "anything else is going on".

Feeling Better

At the end of the day, patients come to the doctor for two reasons. They want to understand what is wrong with them, and they want to know how the doctor can help them feel better. In Long COVID, we are much further along in understanding the cause of symptoms than we are at finding a cure. There is an increasing body of literature on treatments that can help, but patients are often bothered by the answers. They got an infection, now they have a brain problem, and the doctor is prescribing Tai chi, or worse, diagnosing depression and just telling them to go get treated. Some doctors may seem dismissive when they do it, but deep down they know they have little to offer at the moment. They did see a recent article about Tai chi is giving patients significant improvement in quality of life in Long COVID. They may not have read the full article, but the abstract was quite convincing.

The reality is that treatment of cognition is often based on two principles. The first is to optimize whole body health, treating all of the active medical conditions that could each have a small impact on the brain's overall processing speed. This could be treating your diabetes a little more aggressively, doing more to manage depression, or finally getting into a regular diet/exercise routine. The second principle is best summed up by an old famous story. A man was under a lamp post looking around the ground. Another man approaches and asks what he is doing. The first man says he is looking for his keys. The second man offers to help and says, "Are you sure you dropped them here?" The first man says, "No, but this is where the light is." The moral to the story: we treat the things we can identify and know how to treat.

The scientific literature has expanded our understanding of human biology, the abnormal responses the immune system can have to a virus, how that can impact bodily functions, and how all this affects brain activity. However brilliant this light is, it is no more than a lamp post in a large open field. We can choose to fret over the unknown or pretend it does not exist. Alternatively, we can use the data we do have to test for, identify, and treat different conditions that contribute to symptoms. This approach can lead to hope, even though it is not as satisfying as a simple lab test used to diagnose a bacterial infection and treating with an antibiotic, or testing a vitamin level as low and supplementing it. We have no lab test for Long COVID, no MRI for brain fog, but once we can accept that as a reality we can begin to treat the patient and improve quality of life and functional outcomes by treating the components rather than the disease. In this book, I will stay focused on where the light is rather than opine about the unlit areas.

CHAPTER 4: WHAT'S HAPPENING IN MY HEAD?

One of the most common manifestations during and after COVID infection is migraine. However, many patients and even physicians, do not truly understand how much of the post-COVID syndrome is simply a part of classic migraine. In truth, migraine is not really a headache disorder. Migraine is a brain network disorder resulting in difficulty with sensory processing. The whole process starts with a cascade of chemicals beginning with dopamine, deep in the brain, that leads to central sensitization (amplification of sensory signals). This affects the trigeminal nerve that processes all sensory input from most of the head including the skin around the brain (called the meninges). In this way, a variety of types of head pain can occur. However, this is only one of the downstream effects of these chemical changes deep in the brain.

Migraine is one of the most diverse brain disorders with regards to symptom manifestation. Symptoms can come in any combination and tend to fluctuate and evolve over time as the rest of the body changes. This can lead to an enormous amount of confusion for patients who have a misunderstanding of what migraine is. They know they have migraines, but "this is different". Helping patients understand "this is different" is the part of the migraine syndrome that is usually the first and most difficult barrier to getting them treatment.

So, before I talk about why Long COVID is in large part evolution of or development of a migraine syndrome, I should talk a little about the wide world of migraine. Keep in mind that nearly all of migraine relates in some way to sensory processing in the brain.

Severe Head Pain

Why not start with pain? In many patients it is the most debilitating component, though not always. One irony is that head pain is the most likely symptom to cause patients to believe they have a more "serious brain problem" like a tumor, inflammation, or a build up of pressure within the head. This is ironic because, of the many symptoms that come with migraine, it is the least likely to be caused by a "scary" brain disease. The reason for this is obvious: there are no pain receptors in the brain. Most people have heard about or seen videos of brain surgeries performed with the patient wide awake the whole time. Patients are under anesthesia (and/or strong local anesthetics) when neurosurgeons cut the scalp, make a hole in the skull, and open up the meninges, but after that is done surgeons can poke, cut, and zap the brain without the patient feeling a thing. If they use an electrode on the motor areas, the arm may twitch. If they zap the sensory area for the hand, patients may feel tingling in the hand, but they do not feel the brain.

There are some caveats to this. The larger blood vessels in the brain have some sensory fibers in them so a spasming blood vessel can cause pretty severe pain, though not always. A condition called RCVS (reversible cerebral vasoconstriction syndrome) is a headache syndrome where the blood vessels in the brain begin having trouble regulating blood flow. The main symptom that brings folks to the hospital is "recurrent thunderclap headache". A thunderclap headache is where you go from having no headache at all to the "worst headache of your life" within about 5 seconds. It does not worsen from there, but will gradually improve over minutes to hours. The pain can be of nearly any quality, but it is almost always severe enough to send people to the emergency department (ED). ED docs may not know about RCVS because they have been taught that a thunderclap headache is associated with a ruptured aneurysm, which is ok because the evaluation is very similar.

They start with a CT scan of the head to look for blood and then a CT angiogram of the head and neck to look for aneurysms (which is the first set of tests in RCVS to look for spasming blood vessels). If those are normal and the headache goes away, then RCVS is not an emergency. If the headache keeps happening, you will come right back to the emergency department and they should ask a neurologist to help, and the neurologist will know all about RCVS.

It was always known that ischemic strokes do not cause headaches, but that is not entirely true. Ischemic stroke, where a clot closes off a blood vessel and brain tissue dies, almost always comes with a headache, but it is usually pretty mild. When you cannot move your arm because of a stroke, you will not be too worried about the mild headache that comes with it. There are some other pretty serious conditions that do come with headache, but again, the headache is not the serious part and definitely not the main symptom.

Tumors can cause headaches in a few ways. The most common way is by increasing the pressure in your head by blocking drainage of the cerebrospinal fluid. A tumor that bad, or that poorly placed, will have all kinds of other symptoms. If it is at the main drainage areas, it will cause you to be extremely tired, it will be slowly progressive, and it will cause an enormous amount of confusion. You will be coming to the ED for those reasons, not the headache. Some tumors get so big they squish the brain (and the skin around the brain), but then you have all kinds of other brain symptoms (like loss of consciousness) and it is very very slowly progressive and never feels better. Infections and other causes of inflammation can also cause a pretty severe headache that approximates migraine (from meningitis) but again, it is the confusion and other signs of brain damage that usually bring you to the ED, not the headache alone.

When severe headache is a predominant symptom, even with classic episodes, patients inevitably worry the most about getting a brain scan to look for "something else" to explain their symptoms. As a neurologist, headache is often reassuring to me when patients come in with all the atypical perceptual symptoms because it is less likely to be a seizure, tumor, or inflammation if there is a prominent headache. With Long COVID, a neurologist is likely the best physician to get a history, do a physical exam, and confirm if the headache syndrome and the perceptual disturbance is a classic migraine syndrome or something else. With the number of patients developing Long COVID, and the high percentage of them involving the development of a migraine syndrome (over 50%), this is becoming a very common patient concern.

Some people are under the impression that migraine means severe head pain, but from my experience and the experience of many others, it is not the severity of the headache, but the quality, location, and associated features that identify a headache as migrainous.

To explain this, I will describe the other common primary headache syndromes (often more severe than migraine head pain) that may or may not be "mixed" with migraine but do not really respond to migraine treatments. Some of these are also common in Long COVID, but most are extraordinarily rare to occur due to Long COVID. Identifying them is key in making sure "nothing else is going on" and the exam and history are far more important than any blood test or MRI.

Muscular Headache

Muscle/tendon/arthritis pain is a plague on our society, and headache from muscle pain is the most common headache type. At least half of the people referred to my clinic for "headache" have isolated primary tension headaches. Of the other half, maybe 2/3 of them have both migraines and tension headaches. There is a lot of stigma against being diagnosed with tension headaches for a few reasons. Some doctors call them "stress headaches", which introduces societal stigma against psychological components such as anxiety. The word "tension" can also have negative associations. Either way, patients feel far less validated when they "only have a tension headache" and they were sure they had a tumor or an aneurysm. However, while migraines are more debilitating than tension headaches because of the light sensitivity, the fatigue, and the other symptoms, in my migraine patients, often the most painful headaches they have are tension related. Unfortunately, the medications we use for migraines often have a very limited effect on tension predominant headaches.

The textbook says a tension headache is a band around the head, but that is just not true. I have had patients with tension headaches that felt like a deep throb in the side of the head (the textbook description of a migraine) when the main problem was TMJ or a high cervical strain. Tension headaches often include or originate as pain in the neck, and they can range from mild to extremely severe. As a neurologist, my tools have very limited effect on these headaches, though some of my medications are a little more effective than others. Topiramate seems to have a benefit, though no one really knows why. Amitriptyline can help, usually because it helps relax someone while they sleep, allowing the strained muscle(s) to heal. Otherwise, most patients benefit from a treatment plan that combines some form of physical therapy and psychotherapy designed to relax and realign the musculature. Between sleeplessness, muscle fatigue, emotional stress, and neck pain, muscle tension headaches are quite common in Long COVID

Neuralgia

Neuralgiform headaches are another type of headache

that PCPs and patients are curious about. I find them to be a relatively small percentage of my headache referrals, and the reports of their frequency in the general population are very difficult to interpret. Under strict definitions, they are quite rare compared to most other headache types. However, if a research study includes all people with "tenderness" on the back of the head, or some other physician uses that definition, patients may be diagnosed with occipital neuralgia (ON) at very high rates when the real problem is muscle tension. While I do not know any physicians who would intentionally design their diagnosis around higher levels of billing, there are other subtle motivations to diagnose occipital neuralgia. It has an easy procedure that dramatically improves symptoms. A small injection of a numbing agent and a steroid at the spot where the occipital nerve leaves the skull is a wonderful solution for occipital neuralgia. Unfortunately, when patients "feel a little better" after the injection, some providers congratulate themselves for diagnosing an atypical presentation of occipital neuralgia and do not find out from the patient until months later (if ever) that it only helped for a few hours or days. Most of those are tension headaches because of tightness in the muscle next to the nerve.

Neuralgiform headaches can be atypical, but they nearly always have most of the classic features. The quality of the pain is zapping, electrical, burning, or sometimes reported as stabbing. Deep aching or throbbing would be atypical. These headaches should follow a very consistent distribution. The occipital nerve always comes out by that notch on the back of your head (one on each side) and gives sensory information for the scalp nearly to the hair line. If it is compressed or inflamed it does not also come with neck pain or pain on the side of the head. The Trigeminal nerve has three branches which may not all be affected, but trigeminal neuralgia (TGN) is typically very consistent regarding the distribution and may be in the mouth (sometimes including the teeth). If the pain is on the back of the head, and in the neck, and on the side of the face, it is clearly not an individual nerve being affected, making neuralgia unlikely.

Lastly, in addition to a particular type of pain and a particular distribution of the pain, the pain can almost always be caused or worsened by tapping the root of the nerve (just in front of the ear for TGN and on the occipital ridge for ON) with each tap causing a lightning bolt down the nerve. Sometimes these nerves are compressed by small tumors or blood vessel loops, so your doctor may order imaging, but typically these syndromes are from reactive inflammation. This is thought to be in response to a viral or bacterial infection (much less commonly a primary autoimmune condition) where the immune system's response also causes inflammation to attack the nerve.

Some researchers have obsessed over these (and

other neuropathies) being caused by specific viruses like herpes, but research has shown that many different types of infections can cause the same nerve irritation and even damage. This could include scalp and skin infections, ear infections, dental and other oral infections, and often infections throughout the body (upper respiratory or GI). Consequently, specific antiviral treatments and anti-bacterial treatments do not seem to have much effect unless there is evidence of a particular virus. There are many different herpes viruses, but skin herpes and herpes zoster (Shingles) are ones that seem to respond well to antiviral medications. So, in the rare case of a neuralgia headache of the face where there is also a rash on the face or in the ear, antivirals may be helpful, but generally they are not. Steroids can be quite helpful in some cases of nerve inflammation if caught very quickly. Nerve pain is treated with specific types of medication and identifying these less common syndromes can be very important.

Long COVID research has shown that people may develop nerve inflammation in many ways. There are cases of Bell's Palsy (dysfunction to the nerve for the face muscles), Guillain-Barre syndrome (dysfunction of the longer nerves in the body), and small fiber neuropathy (dysfunction or damage to the small nerves in the skin) after COVID infection. This would indicate that either the post-acute sequelae of COVID or the Long COVID syndrome could have other common post-viral nerve inflammation components like Occipital or Trigeminal neuralgia. However, specific prevalence data is unclear. I personally have had a few patients develop a neuralgia headache either during COVID, after COVID, or after vaccination for COVID, but they were mild cases that were easy to treat.

So, increased pressure in the head, infections, tension headaches, and nerve pain headaches can all be identified more by the other symptoms than the location of the pain or the severity, but the most common post-COVID headache is migraine. This may involve severe pain or mild pain and can have features of other headache types, but fundamentally, migraine is a sensory processing disorder so the headache has some unique features.

Sensory Sensitivities

Migraine headaches are significantly impacted by all senses. While many types of pain can be "blinding" if severe, if a headache is dramatically affected by light, sound, or smell, that is much more consistent with migraine. Dizziness and nausea are similar. Any pain can cause nausea or dizziness if it is very severe, but if the dizziness or nausea is an early and prominent feature, migraine is more likely. As mentioned above, most of the pain signal in migraine comes from a sensitivity of the trigeminal nerve signals from the skin around the brain, the meninges. The trigeminal nerve also supplies the face, so people may have "sensitivity" of the skin of the face or scalp causing pain with light touch, a phenomenon known as allodynia.

Migraineurs may say their hair hurts, they can't wear their glasses, or they can't touch the skin because it feels like a sunburn, numb, or tender. These sensory symptoms are called paresthesias or allodynia and they mostly occur on the head, but can also be experienced in other nerve distributions. It is unclear how much of this is due to the brain processing a normal signal differently (due to central sensitization) or the nerves being over activated (peripheral sensitization), but it is likely a combination of both. If a bad headache is associated with arm tingling, I feel much more confident it is migraine. Arm tingling could be a pinched nerve or even seizure activity, but that would not lead to a bad headache. A bad headache can be caused by a thousand medical problems, but if it comes with feeling your arm has a sunburn, it is almost always a migraine. If you had some visual disturbances or it seemed to be caused by lights around you, those combinations make migraine far more likely and more scary diagnoses less likely. A very large percentage of my Long COVID patients have these symptoms occur both during the headache and also when they are not having a headache. Those symptoms are almost always responsive to migraine medications and treatments, and are only very rarely associated with other medical conditions.

So, the pain is possibly the least useful way to define migraine, but the other symptoms along with headache of nearly any quality or severity are quite helpful. These symptoms can occur in the absence of head pain as well, and that can lead to some of the strangest, most frightening, and most often misdiagnosed migraines. I will now discuss those other potential symptoms based on their causes, patterns, and other features.

Dizziness

The most common feature of migraine, when not properly treated, involves complex processing of sensory information. As mentioned before, at its core, migraine is a sensory processing disorder. Sometimes this involves hypersensitivity to an individual sensation (light or sound sensitivity) even in the absence of a headache, but often the symptom is due to difficulty putting sensations together properly. Dizziness is likely the most common "symptom" in this category.

Dizziness is a very difficult word in medicine. For one person, dizziness is a feeling of lightheadedness, like when you're dehydrated or on too many blood pressure meds. You stand up, you get a wave of dizziness and feel you might faint. For another person, dizziness is room spinning. There are a few classic causes of vertigo, where the signal from the inner ear is misbehaving. Your eyes are telling you that you are still, but your ear is sending a signal that your head is turning (or vice versa). The world seems to spin around you, or you seem to spin around the world. These classic causes of vertigo are pretty easy to diagnose with a good timeline and a quick exam, but vertigo is still very often misdiagnosed or misunderstood by patients and primary care doctors.

The Three Vertigos

The most common type of vertigo is benign paroxysmal positional vertigo (BPPV). In BPPV, very small "crystals" build up in the little organs of the inner ear and change the way fluid moves. This consequently causes a bad signal to the brain. It is easy to identify because the same movement can cause the symptom every time. You turn to your left or sit up in a certain way and it consistently causes a brief wave of spinning that resolves pretty quickly if you keep your head still. On exam, I can cause the symptom with a dix-hallpike maneuver and, more importantly, can see very specific changes to your eye movements (nystagmus). It works every time and the sensation is always accompanied by the eye movements (unless you have taken medication to blunt the signals). The treatment is to do a different more complex maneuver called the "Epley" designed to make the crystals fall out of that part of the inner ear. Often you must do the procedure frequently until the symptoms no longer occur because where there is one crystal there are often many more. It is called paroxysmal because the crystals can build up again if you are dehydrated, just like people who are predisposed to kidney stones or gallstones.

Another common condition is called vestibular neuritis (or labyrinthitis if another organ is involved). This often occurs after an infection and is very similar to the neuritis I mentioned above, and we often give steroids for the same reason if we catch it early. It is caused by inflammation of the vestibular nerve or parts of the inner ear and it has a very classic history with a very classic exam. In this case, it ramps up over a day or two, lasts a few weeks, and gradually improves. This is a pretty nasty syndrome and people feel terrible. Keeping your head still usually does not help much, but moving makes it worse, so people typically stay quite still when they are not falling down and vomiting. Looking to one direction (either right or left depending on the affected ear) will make you feel much better and looking the opposite will make you feel like you might die because you are so dizzy. Otherwise, it does not change too much during the course of the illness. Apart from steroids if you catch it early, there is not much else to be done besides rest and taking medications to mask the symptoms until the course of the illness resolves (over a few weeks).

The third cause of spinning dizziness that is not uncommon is called Meniere's disease. Again, a relatively classic syndrome caused by changes to fluid in the inner ear. It often occurs as a triad of symptoms (remember chapter 1?) including hearing loss or severe tinnitus, pain in the ear, and debilitating room spinning vertigo similar to the experience of vestibular neuritis. Luckily, this syndrome lasts only a few hours per spell for most patients and not multiple weeks, but it can be quite frequent and debilitating. The main treatments are reducing salt intake, adding diuretics, or procedures performed by ear nose and throat docs.

While I have had a number of patients develop a primary vertigo after COVID, it does not seem to be a common or primary symptom of Long COVID. At times, the vestibular neuritis or labyrinthitis has occurred, but they are usually during or immediately after the COVID-19 infection, just like it occurs during or right after any other infection. In most cases of BPPV and Meniere's disease after COVID, they already had a history of those types of spells. BPPV or Meniere's recurrence is often due to dehydration and other stressors on the body. The main cause of dizziness genuinely due to Long COVID is a dizziness associated with migraine that has a lot to do with migraine's sensory processing disturbances.

Perceptual Dizziness

Dizziness in migraine can have many different features from a rare pure vestibular syndrome (which mimics the room spinning like other vertigos) to a variety of components of mixed symptoms with lightheadedness, disequilibrium, and room spinning that can range from mildly uncomfortable to debilitating. There may be a subjective room spinning, but often it is more akin to motion sickness like sea sickness or car sickness without being on a boat or in a car. It might have a light headedness component or a discomfort while tracking moving objects. The exam is typically either "normal" neurologically or a very specific finding where dizziness can be caused by eye movements regardless of head movement. There is a related syndrome that is more common in migraineurs and is associated with untreated vertigo called persistent postural perceptual dizziness. It may be persistent outside of "migraine episodes" and is treated with simple antidepressants (SSRIs) and vestibular therapy.

Distinct spells of dizziness are common components of migraine and have a specific cause in the brain called "cortical spreading depression" (CSD). It could be considered the opposite of seizure activity. In seizure, electrical activity ramps up and organizes causing an increase in energy requirement for an area of brain tissue. In CSD there is a slowing of brain activity with a reduction in energy use. It will usually start in one area of the brain and spread along networks like seizure activity and can consequently have many similar features. Fundamentally, CSD is the core cause of most of the "very weird" symptoms that are associated with migraine. Why this happens is not fully understood, and it is impossible to give a full accounting of the variety of symptoms potentially caused by CSD. If they occur for around 20 minutes, typically before a migraine headache, they are called an aura. I find they can occur just as often separated from the headache spells, during the headache spells, or after the headache spells. Because migraine is so common in Long COVID, the majority of COVID related dizziness I see is part of the migraine related persistent postural perceptual dizziness syndrome.

Cortical Spreading Depression

When CSD occurs in or around the primary visual cortex, it leads to the classic visual aura. Sparkling lights, zig zag lines, rainbow squiggles, and spots in the vision (like if you stare at a bright light and then look away) are quite common. When they spread to the visual association cortex, it can lead to visual distortions of many kinds that are collectively referred to as Alice in Wonderland syndrome. Perhaps the room grows around you or people shrink. Maybe just their head gets big or small. Nearby areas of the brain process spatial movement and even time perception leading to feeling as if time or space dilates, losing track of how long something is occurring, how close objects are, or how fast something is moving.

If the CSD occurs in the sensory processing areas of the brain, many types of sensation can occur. This includes tingling, numbness, burning, zapping, or sensitivity to touch. It is often worse on one side and can fluctuate similarly to the other CSD symptoms. Usually there is not anesthesia of the skin, where if you touch the skin the sensation of light touch is diminished, but that can occur at times as well. I have heard patients describe a throbbing, a vibration sensation, wetness, fullness, and many other types of sensory disturbances collectively referred to as paresthesias. Likewise, people can have this happen to the motor areas of the brain leading to feelings of weakness.

Moving into the temporal lobe, people can have prolonged Deja Vu, out of body experiences, and even ecstatic or frightening experiences that could be interpreted as spiritual. This is not unlike how scientists believe Joan of Arc had epileptic seizures in the temporal lobe leading to visions of God. People can have major changes to language perception if the CSD hits the language areas of the brain, extreme emotional reactions if it moves into the limbic region, or vivid daydreams and hallucinations if it moves into other areas. Since it is opposite of seizure, it will often have some differences in quality and typically causes less severe brain dysfunction, but since all areas that can seize can also have CSD, there is a large amount of overlap. All of this can happen when the Long COVID syndrome includes a prominent migraine component.

Other Migraine Syndromes

There is another type of syndrome that can occur associated with migraines that is fundamentally a little different and may be more worrisome. It is caused by dysfunction of the brainstem and is quite rare compared to the above syndromes. It is typically associated with a genetic disorder and will often run in families. The two most often described are the "hemiplegic migraine" and the "vestibular migraine". The hemiplegic migraine is very difficult to distinguish from a large stroke. It happens in a very similar way over and over, and is a very pronounced weakness on just one side of the body. The true vestibular migraine is very difficult to distinguish from a brainstem stroke or a primary vertigo. These folks do not always have headaches when they get dizzy spells. They are in the emergency department for severe room spinning that makes the headache practically irrelevant. These sorts of brainstem migraines are associated with an increased risk of stroke, so particular attention needs to be paid to medications. Many medications we use in migraine can cause minor bloodvessel spasming (Triptans, Ergots, SNRIs, and others) and we avoid these medications in true brainstem migraines. Also, women should be very careful not to smoke cigarettes and should try to avoid high dose hormone contraceptive medications.

So, since migraine is one of the most common symptoms in the Long COVID syndrome, all of the above are potential symptoms that could be treated with migraine medications and behavioral treatments. I will go into them more thoroughly in the chapters on medications, physical therapies, and behavioral treatments, but a few things should be emphasized about these treatments, their limitations, and the research behind them.

Clinical Considerations

The first thing to know about migraine treatments is the data behind them is very limited. We have used these medications, with very good results, for so long they were not on patent when we discovered their usefulness. Consequently, no large pharmaceutical company would make money off of studying them, and so no large double blind trials have ever been done. There is a LOT of research out there, but typically either in small studies or studies asking a different question. There is no large study for propranolol compared to placebo, but there are a hundred studies comparing propranolol to other therapies and looking at combination treatments. There are studies on amitriptyline showing it helps both with migraine and with other symptoms, or that it is more effective when combined with topiramate, but nothing where amitriptyline was compared to placebo in a large enough trial to guide any changes in how we prescribe it. Also, a trial might just give 25mg and that is not how we prescribe it because patients often need to start lower and their eventual dose depends a lot on how well they tolerate it and how effective it is at different doses. We start at 10mg, increase to 25mg, and then increase further if there are benefits but not enough to really resolve the problem.

Another limitation of the data regarding migraine treatments is that very few people study the non-headache components of migraine. Headaches are easy to track. Someone can report 16 headaches in 30 days and give each a 0-10 severity. But how do you give a number to fatigue, dizziness, or visual distortions? How do you give a numerical value to light sensitivity? It has always been expert opinion that the other symptoms of migraine tend to respond to medications similarly to headache, but we do not have good data to confirm. Maybe amitriptyline is better for allodynia than topiramate. Maybe venlafaxine is better for migraine associated dizziness than propranolol. Many neurologists have noticed patterns based on their own predisposition as phenomenologists, but the assumption is limited by a lack of research and the difficulty of studying more subjective symptoms. Again, you would be better served by a physician using a standard algorithm for treating migraine than someone calling it an infection and using disproven or experimental treatments. However, you may want to ask follow up questions about different medication options and why your neurologist or primary care physician would recommend one over another.

As with many topics in human medicine, patients learning about migraine should avoid random Google search results or looking at non-moderated online groups. There are a few conditions in neurology where I actually recommend the patient google it so they can see how benign it is. Transient Global Amnesia is a terribly frightening condition to patients until they do a quick search and see how benign it is. Meralgia Paresthetica is a very common cause of leg numbness that is the same from patient to patient and googling it may help reduce fear that a more dangerous condition is being "missed". But as I have described above, migraine is extremely complex and symptom combinations differ from person to person. Searching online will often lead patients to articles by 1% of migraine patients where a disaster occurred, or many articles from writers who do not really understand the condition.

Conclusions

At the end of the day, learning how your brain can misbehave due to Long COVID related migraine requires an individualized approach with close monitoring by a neurologist you trust. Migraines evolve over time by nature, can lead to a thousand clinical symptoms, and can be terrifying. However, potentially more dangerous is when new symptoms are ignored because a patient becomes sensitized to strange perceptual experiences. Having migraines does not protect a patient from having strokes, seizures, inflammatory disorders, or other serious and treatable conditions. Obsessing over symptoms or ignoring them can lead to major trouble.

I always tell my patients there is never a scenario where they must worry alone. I ask them to let me worry with them, and to travel with them expecting bumps and turns along the road. The more I know them and their baseline symptoms and exam, the more I can confidently assure them that a new symptom should not be a source of worry. Likewise, I may find a change in their physical neurologic exam that might guide further workup or a different treatment. However I present the information, problems occur if my patients hear in my words or my tone of voice that their distress is not justified and nothing is wrong with them, that their symptom is "only migraine". If that happens, they will often not return to me for follow-up exams or when they have a new symptom. I see this as a failing on my part, and strive to make sure patients know that they are heard and that their symptoms and distress is taken seriously.

So if you are a neurologist (or any physician really), make sure you get your patient's perspective on what is wrong at each visit in their own words. Try not to diminish their suffering by saying that their problem is "only migraine". Emphasize that when there is a new symptom it might make you do further workup or consider other treatments. Let them know that you will adapt as their symptoms adapt and that you will treat each case as a unique one, even if it seems textbook at first. I have had dozens of textbook migraine patients with sensory disturbances turn into textbook multiple sclerosis or another inflammatory condition. Likewise, I have had textbook multiple sclerosis turn into textbook sarcoidosis. The textbook is a limited guideline for where to start based on a snapshot in time. If your patients understand you will change course with new information rather than anchoring on a previous theory, they will come back. Otherwise, they will go see someone else, delaying identification of a new problem, creating redundant workups that exhaust our healthcare system, and perpetuating a message that they are alone in their struggle and worsening their medical trauma.

And if you are a patient, keep faith and keep searching for a provider you can trust, regardless of if your symptoms are Long COVID related. Perhaps your trusted physician is a primary care doctor who can translate the note by the specialist and recommend a second opinion when it makes sense. Maybe you have a general neurologist but want a specialist for a new and specific question, with a plan to return to that general neurologist after the specialist is done evaluating your weakness or pain. Keep looking for someone you can trust and do not let them go. Also be wary of anyone who "definitely knows what's wrong" with you, but insists it isn't their job to treat you. It is inappropriate for a neurologist at a big academic center to tell you that you need very specific therapy for a rare disorder, but insist that another neurologist or provider prescribe it. Sure, your neurologist may ask your PCP to be in charge of pain management, or to try first line treatments before sending you back to a specialist for a common condition, but it is important to centralize your care so that you have a team you will trust to ease your worries, and who you trust to worry for you when it is necessary. This is especially true with a condition as complex, multifaceted, distressing, and treatable as Long COVID related migraine.

CHAPTER 5: IS THERE A PILL FOR THIS?

General Considerations

Books could be written on each and every medication I consider in Long COVID, and there are too many potential options to put into this one chapter. However, I always try to remind patients and their physicians there are many potential tools at our disposal. Unfortunately, one size most definitely does not fit all. In an ideal world, especially with medications that can affect mood, a patient would have very frequent follow-ups with both a therapist and a psychiatrist to help monitor the effects. There can be subtle changes in depression, mania, perception, and sensory symptoms that are not expected when initiating medications. Psychotherapy can help patients predict and understand these experiences as well as monitor patients for benefits and side effects. This can improve a sense of well being despite uncomfortable, but temporary, side effects.

It is important to understand that research is done on populations and I have only treated individuals. Rare side effects can occur, but analyzing the risks for an individual can be impossible because of the way these studies are designed. Common effects can also offset each other. If half of the patients gain 10 lbs and the other half lose 10 lbs, the study may show weight changes are unlikely, even if they are almost inevitable. Also, while most patients tolerate the initial plan to start low and increase slowly to a high dose, I always tell patients that we may have to go slower if side effects occur. "Pushing through" side effects can be a good plan, but only to a point. Before starting these medications it is key to discuss expectations and potential plans to adjust. This can help prevent discomfort and, in rare cases, disaster.

Below I will discuss some of the major categories and common medications that have been studied in chronic fatigue syndrome, its individual symptoms, and my preferred method of escalation and monitoring. I do not, however, claim these are the right ways or the only ways to prescribe these medications and in some cases, I change the plan based on the patient in front of me. I list the most common side effects I see in clinical practice, but your prescriber should familiarize themselves with any up to date warnings or monitoring protocols. I find that when patients have "failed" these medications in the past, one of two problems occurred: 1. they started at too high of a dose and tolerate it better with a "start low, go slow" model, or 2. the medication was abandoned at too low of a dose that is not expected to have much of an effect. Also, primary care doctors may have previously used these medications with a different escalation protocol designed to treat different conditions. They may not know to start lower or to increase higher in patients with Long COVID, chronic fatigue, and migraine. Often prescribers may be overly safe, delaying benefit, or overly aggressive, causing discomfort, but these medications are ultimately very safe and patients' fears are typically out of proportion to the risk.

Melatonin

Melatonin is considered to be generally safe in most patients at a very broad dosing range. Benefits can occur at very low doses like 0.5 mg and can increase safely with use up to 20mg or more. It is not a classical sedative, and has very little effect on breathing or other bodily functions. Some people take it as needed, but it is typically better used daily because it works by signaling to the brain that it is night time. The brain makes its own melatonin, which increases into the evening and reduces into the morning, as part of the sleep-wake cycle. It is also very quickly eliminated from the body so that within 1 hour most of it has been metabolized. Patients may still feel groggy in the morning, but it is not because the melatonin lasts that long. The grogginess from melatonin is likely because the brain is actually getting into a deep sleep and does not want to wake up. While this is the main mechanism of melatonin, there are many possible actions throughout the body. Melatonin receptors are found on the pancreas, liver, kidney, heart, lung, fat, and intestinal tissues. It may have an important role in hormones and glands during fetal development, but there is not any data to suggest these are relevant in adults.

I recommend taking this medicine at the exact same time every night as part of a winding down ritual. There is no wrong dose to start at, but I usually recommend 1mg nightly for a week and then increase to 3mg nightly, 5mg nightly, and then 10mg nightly each week that no major difference is noted. It can either be taken around sundown, or an hour before bedtime. There are other, newer, medications that work on the melatonin system, but I have yet to see any data to suggest they are mechanistically different even though they may be considered stronger and are more expensive.

Serotonin Based Medications

These medications were originally designed as antidepressants due to a theory of how serotonin affects mood. This has been hotly debated, and I can comfortably say that the more we understand serotonin's effects on the brain, the less we understand how these medications affect depression. However, we are learning more about how they support networks related to thought, sensory processing, and reactivity to both internal and external stimuli. While these medications are deemed very safe, the patient must be monitored frequently for manic symptoms, especially if they have a family history. In some cases, an EKG is important to confirm there is no heart rhythm abnormality. Lastly, combining them or using them at high doses in some people may cause a condition called Serotonin Syndrome. This syndrome can lead to diarrhea, panic, muscle rigidity, and other autonomic symptoms like sweating or inability to sweat and can be life threatening if supportive treatment is delayed.

Tricyclics (amitriptyline, nortriptyline, and others)

Originally used for anxiety and depression as well as other psychiatric conditions, currently the vast majority of prescribed tricyclics are used for chronic pain or migraine. There are some subtle differences between them, but they share the same list of possible effects and side effects. The goal, as always in neurology, is to use the side effects to help other symptoms or to use one medication for dual purposes. For this reason, tricyclic medications are often the best choice when used in patients with migraine or chronic pain who also suffer from insomnia since drowsiness is a common side effect. Amitriptyline, for example, was once used at doses of 150mg and even as high as 300mg nightly in some cases of depression, but in migraine and insomnia quite small doses (25mg or 50mg) can have a dramatic impact over time in reducing spells. Similar dosing can also help chronic pain from many other conditions. It works by strengthening the brain networks in charge of reducing the pain signal, and the extra sleep does not hurt. Doctors might choose clomipramine (a similar drug) at higher doses if they are also trying to treat specific disorders like panic syndrome or obsessive compulsive syndrome at the same time. Side effects vary widely, with dry mouth, some weight gain, and morning drowsiness being the most common, but for most patients the side effects at low doses resolve within a week or two.

I recommend starting with amitriptyline 10mg nightly for 2 weeks and then increasing to 20mg nightly for 2-4 weeks until I meet with patients to monitor side effects and benefits. Starting at bedtime is reasonable, but if there is a "hungover" feeling in the morning after a few days, they should advance the dose earlier in the day until the hungover feeling goes away or they feel too drowsy too early. If they do not adapt quickly to this I will switch to the equal dose of nortriptyline, which usually does not cause morning drowsiness. Some physicians start with nortriptyline, but I do not find it quite as effective. I typically slowly increase to between 50-100mg and rarely go up to 200mg in cases where we continue to get benefit.

SSRIs

While there is some data to suggest that SSRIs can help with chronic fatigue, migraine, and chronic pain, the data is less clear than with other medications. They have also been most well studied in Persistent Postural Perceptual Dizziness previously discussed. SSRIs can help activate those frontal brain networks which cause depression-like symptoms, but for any individual symptom (fatigue, drowsiness, low energy, brain fog, pain) they are not as predictable. Sertraline is particularly useful because it can be started at a very low dose and increased over time to treat different symptoms at different doses, including obsessive/compulsive symptoms at very high doses (>200mg daily). Fluoxetine is great when someone has a hard time remembering to take the medication every day because it takes about a month to wash out of your system, so accidental withdrawal symptoms are unlikely. While most people tolerate each SSRI very well, individuals may rarely have release of suicidal thoughts, feeling like a zombie, etc. These concerns often go away after being on a stable dose for a while. However, because of potential release of suicidal thinking and mania, these medicines should be very closely monitored by a therapist and/or psychiatrist during initiation.

Obviously the choice of which SSRI to use can have many considerations, but I typically start with sertraline at a low dose and slowly increase it to effect. I start at 25mg daily for 2 weeks (switching to nightly dosing if drowsiness is a side effect). Then I increase to

50mg daily for a month, then 100mg for 2 weeks, then 150mg for a month, and then 200mg if symptoms have not resolved or side effects have not occurred. If obsessive thoughts are present I will then go to 250mg and then to 300mg, waiting there for at least 2 months before changing the plan. Escitalopram and Citalopram are very well tolerated in many people, but typically have a much smaller dosing range and seem to have more hard ceilings for the dose due to heart rhythm concerns limiting continued escalation for continued benefits. Citalopram is especially difficult in older adults because the guidelines say it should not go above 20mg in older individuals (40mg in younger patients). Paroxetine is very complex, has a much higher likelihood of side effects and interactions, and is probably best avoided. However, some patients have a uniquely good response to it for depression symptoms so it cannot be forgotten entirely.

SNRIs

Like SSRIs, these medications can treat depression (or depression-like symptoms), but they also have a variety of other benefits. At higher doses, they can also reduce migraine/chronic pain. Duloxetine is very well tolerated, like SSRIs, and has a similar side effect profile. Venlafaxine is considered to be more "activating", leading to improvements in concentration and reduced forgetfulness in many patients. It can be difficult to use in patients with high blood pressure, but in patients who faint from a drop in blood pressure (POTS syndrome, or lightheadedness seen in Long COVID) it can reduce light headedness and dizziness. It is also considered more weight neutral (less likely to cause weight gain). Unfortunately, there is less data on safety at higher doses due to all of these other effects, so we cannot increase to doses that would better treat OCD symptoms. SNRIs are also more likely to cause unpredictable, but typically non-dangerous side effects in patients who have physical anxiety symptoms (stomach discomfort, heart racing, lump in the throat, etc). A third SNRI, L-milnacepran, is mostly used just for chronic pain, but it is prescribed less often for mood so clinical experience is more limited.

Venlafaxine is typically my first choice for an SNRI in Long COVID. I start at 37.5mg extended release daily and increase to 75mg daily after 2 weeks if well tolerated. After 4 weeks at 75mg I discuss how well it is helping and any side effects before going right to 150mg and staying there for at least a month. The true benefits of norepinephrine are not seen until getting to 150 mg - 225 mg, so I typically try to get the patient to the full dose if they are doing ok at 150mg. Rarely, I have had to reduce back to 150mg due to side effects, or (after a repeat EKG) increase to 300mg to get more benefit. Duloxetine is a wonderful medication and can be more well tolerated than venlafaxine in many patients. It is less "activating" in many, and it is more likely to cause weight gain, but it can help in very similar ways. I typically start with 20mg twice daily and increase slowly, once monthly on average, going up to 60mg twice daily.

Adrenaline System Medications

The adrenaline system is very involved in most of the symptoms of Long COVID, from sleep cycle regulation to fatigue to heart rate and even breathing. There are many ways to modify the adrenaline system, but the benefits and drawbacks sometimes offset each other. Stimulants may help fatigue and brain fog but worsen mania, panic, heart rate, and migraine. Adrenaline blocking treatments may help uncomfortable anxiety symptoms, migraine, and heart rate, but worsen feelings of fatigue and brain fog. While these medications are typically quite safe and have few side effects when they are the right medication, it can take some trials and setbacks to find the right options for an individual patient.

Propranolol

This medicine blocks one of the many adrenaline receptors, and was originally used as a blood pressure treatment. Lightheadedness is one of the main side effects that doctors worry about, but in young healthy people who have lightheadedness because of a fast heart rate (POTS and Long COVID) it can often stabilize blood pressure. Primary care doctors and cardiologists rarely use it anymore because there are many other options without activity in the brain, but for migraine and POTS the goal is to block the adrenaline receptors in the brain. We now use this medicine for migraine, atypical fainting or lightheadedness, and tremor almost exclusively. Side effects can be seen based on how much adrenaline you use for each daily activity. For people who really run on adrenaline, this medicine can cause fatigue or even depression-like symptoms. Living on adrenaline is unhealthy, so this is good information and can help guide other methods (often non-medicine based) to regulate energy such as working on sleep quality, nutrition, and self care.

Prazosin

Being chronically sick or limited is traumatic enough. Additionally, research shows that early life trauma or severe trauma affects the immune system, the adrenaline system, and the brain networks for threat perception. This can predispose to chronic pain processing and chronic fatigue in conditions like Long COVID. Prazosin was originally a blood pressure medication that works on a different adrenaline receptor (alpha 1) than propranolol and has some uniquely beneficial effects. Mainly, it helps sleep by reducing severe nightmares from PTSD. It does not have any unique usefulness in Long COVID, but I have cared for dozens of patients where nightmares and poor sleep quality greatly affect their fatigue, and prazosin was a major part of their care. It does not get rid of nightmares, but it does reduce the adrenaline response, so that patients do not wake in a panic and spend an hour settling back down.

Prazosin is typically started at 1mg nightly and increased every few days to 2mg, 3mg, 5mg, 7mg, and 10mg over the course of a few months as tolerated to limit lightheadedness. If patients have daily hypervigilance or constant subtle panic symptoms, then I will continue to increase it to up to 15mg nightly, then add a 5mg daytime dose, and continue to escalate to up to 30mg total daily dose split with a bigger night time dose (ie: 10mg each morning and 20mg each night). These doses are rarely required and often cannot be reached either because benefits do not increase or side effects do.

Stimulants

Stimulant use in neurology and psychiatry has always been very controversial. They range in strength from caffeine to cocaine, and they all have very similar potential benefits and downsides. There are very strong opinions that they are underused and other strong opinions that they should be used only rarely. The former argue they can be life changing and untreated disorders like ADHD lead to anxiety, depression, and very poor functioning, which can all be effectively treated with stimulants. The opposition argue stimulants can improve focus and productivity in anyone, akin to cocaine, and because the medications help people remain productive it is just a performance enhancing drug. I will not argue either, but to say that fundamentally these are safe medications when prescribed by someone who can monitor them properly. Like many medications in Long COVID, they are helpful for very specific symptoms, but do not change the underlying cause of the problem. They generally improve some of the low-energy/low-mood depression-like symptoms, and they can help with brain fog/forgetfulness. The potential downsides are worsening heart rate disturbances, dependency, hyperactivity and mania, sleep disturbances, and worsening migraine. It must be kept in mind that these are only potential downsides and stimulants can be very safely and effectively used with close monitoring.

"Softer stimulants" can include modafinil, armodafinil, amantadine, and a few new agents almost exclusively used in narcolepsy (solriamfetol, pitolisant). These are generally considered safe alternatives, though they have the exact same list of potential side effects as more traditional stimulants. Amantadine has been particularly well studied in fatigue and cognitive symptoms in a variety of neurologic disorders like multiple sclerosis and Parkinson's. Often, modafinil is a good first choice for these symptoms, but it is not superior or fundamentally safer than the others.

I will typically start modafinil at 100mg daily for 1 week and then increase to 200mg daily until we discuss side effects and benefits. It can go up to 400mg daily. If that is not tolerated or is not effective, I offer to try armodafinil or methylphenidate. If they choose methylphenidate, I always start with small doses of the immediate release until I find a good dose for a patient and then transition to the extended release. At times, patients need an extended release in the morning and an immediate release in the early afternoon to get them through the day, but it is very important to monitor sleep quality because taking a dose later in the day can lead to either insomnia or poor sleep quality, which is absolutely counterproductive. A good starting dose is 10mg in the morning, adding a second 10mg dose as soon as a pattern of "wearing off" is identified. I tell patients to take the second dose about 30 minutes before the expected wearing off. I then increase each dose as tolerated to effect. As soon as a clear benefit with minimal side effects is reached, I switch to the same dose but extended release, which may not feel "quite as effective" at first, but after a few weeks often begins to feel similar to the immediate release. Only after methylphenidate has been shown to have some clear problem or is not effective at high doses, do I transition to more classic amphetamines like adderall. Adderall always feels more effective to patients, but that is usually a pleasure response from the amphetamine and not actually a sign the medication is working properly.

Other Medications

Dopamine Blocking Medications

While stimulants and some antidepressants increase dopamine in the brain, blocking dopamine (only on an as needed basis) can have a very beneficial effect on certain symptoms of migraine. In fact, one of the first chemicals in the brain that misbehaves in the migraine syndrome is dopamine. This is often referred to as the dopamine cascade. The most commonly used dopamine blocking medication in migraine is called metoclopramide (or Reglan), which is typically prescribed for nausea. In some patients the anti-nausea benefit is a huge relief, but blocking dopamine can also help the migraine pain syndrome, the perceptual disturbances, and can help patients fall asleep, which is in and of itself a treatment for migraine. It is even more effective when taken with a small amount of benadryl and a large glass of water, which have a synergistic effect. Benadryl also "cures" the very rare side effect that can occur called a "dystonic reaction". When patients start this type of medication, I recommend keeping a benadryl on hand even if they do not expect to use it in case their neck cramps up or their eyes spasm (called oculogyric crisis). Other medications in this class were designed as mood stabilizers and anti-psychotic treatments. They are extraordinarily helpful when used infrequently in migraine, but have other potential downsides.

I typically recommend starting with metoclopramide 10mg and have patients try it with a half tablet of benadryl (12.5mg) and a large glass of water. It can be safely taken with a triptan or with an NSAID like ibuprofen or naproxen. If 10mg causes drowsiness, I recommend trying 5mg or taking it and laying down for sleep. In patients with >1 week of migraine symptoms, I tend to prescribe olanzapine to abort it, prescribing 2.5mg the first night, 5mg the second night, and increasing each night up to 10mg until it completely resolves the migraine spell. If it has not worked after 7 days, I stop the trial.

Other "Antidepressants"

It is a longstanding debate if mirtazapine is truly an antidepressant. Since we measure depression based on symptom burden, and two of the main symptoms of depression in some (especially older) patients are insomnia and poor appetite, mirtazapine can be very useful. Weight gain is not a side effect of the medicine, but a primary effect. It is a strange medication in that the lowest doses often have the strongest effects on sleep and appetite with higher doses theoretically helping other depression symptoms. It is usually started at 15mg nightly, but I often start even lower at 7.5mg nightly. In some patients, a lower dose is more helpful with fewer non-specific side effects.

Trazodone is also a medication that could theoretically be called an antidepressant. It causes drowsiness at doses between 50mg and 200mg and is universally used as a sleep-aid. I very rarely start it, since the only benefit is sleep and it does not have the side benefits of mirtazapine (improving appetite) or amitriptyline (migraine or chronic pain relief). Since it works on a similar mechanism, I often will transition people to one of the other options, but I have had more than a few patients who did very well when combining trazodone with one of the other options.

Bupropion is a very important option for treatment of depression symptoms in Long COVID, but I do not typically start with it. It works on the dopamine and norepinephrine systems, which can be counterproductive. It can help focus and attention (even being used for ADHD symptoms in some) and it can reduce appetite and other habits like smoking, but it is just as likely to worsen migraine as to help it. However, when added to an SSRI, it will often resolve side effects from the SSRI like weight gain and sexual dysfunction. Technically, adding bupropion to an SSRI like sertraline is kind of like switching to an SNRI like venlafaxine, but if the SSRI is working well then it is a great option.

Mood Stabilizers/Seizure medications

Another group of medications that have particular use in Long COVID are medications that work on settling down nerves by acting on sodium channels, potassium channels, GABA receptors, and other sites. These medications were originally designed for treatment of epilepsy, but they can have remarkable and unique other benefits.

CHAPTER 5: IS THERE A PILL FOR THIS?   119

Topiramate (or alternatively zonisamide) is probably the most common medication I prescribe in this group. It has mild mood stabilizing effects, but we mostly use it for headaches. It helps nearly every type of headache, including increased head pressure headaches. It must be started at a very low dose to reduce side effects. I usually start 25mg nightly for 1 week, then 25mg twice daily for 1 week, and then slowly increase to 50mg twice daily and monitor for effectiveness. We avoid it in people with certain vision problems and/or frequent kidney stones. It can have forgetfulness as a side effect, limiting its use in Long COVID, but it helps with weight loss, reduces urge to snack, smoke, and drink, and when tolerated it can be extraordinarily helpful.

Gabapentin (or alternatively pregabalin) is another medication that has particular usefulness in Long COVID. It can be taken as needed or regularly quite safely to treat some of the chronic pain components. It mostly helps with Neuropathic pain, which is the zappy burny pain. It has a very broad dosing range, between 100mg and 1500mg per dose, up to 3-4 times daily. This dosing schedule can make it inconvenient to start. It is most likely to cause drowsiness and can rarely worsen breathing problems and leg swelling. However, in patients with nerve quality pain, with or without evidence of nerve damage, gabapentin can be a very useful tool.

Similar benefits with variable side effects can

be seen with medications such as oxcarbazepine, carbamazepine, and valproate. Those are sometimes chosen based on an individual side effect benefit and there is not anything unique to Long COVID that guides their use.

Symptoms

Another way to consider treatment is based on which medications (or medication classes) are more likely to help with certain symptoms. It is important to understand the subtleties above, and to understand that treating sleep alone can help nearly all symptoms.

Migraine- Amitriptyline, Venlafaxine, Topiramate, Propranolol, Melatonin

Chronic Aching Pain- Amitriptyline, Venlafaxine

Nerve Pain - Gabapentin, Topiramate, Oxcarbazepine

Dizziness/lightheadedness-   Propranolol,   SNRIs, SSRIs, Tricyclics

Heart racing/fainting- Propranolol, Venlafaxine

Fatigue/brain fog- Venlafaxine, Stimulants

Nausea/poor appetite- Metoclopramide, Mirtazapine

Insomnia- Melatonin, Amitriptyline, Mirtazapine

Immunomodulators

In short, while Long COVID, like Myalgic Encephalomyelitis, is thought to be caused by a dysfunctional immune system (with other contributors for sure), there has been no good data on the prevention or treatment of either condition with the use of immune system modifying drugs. Nevertheless, I would be remiss to leave out a brief narrative and reference to the data we have available.

B-Cell Therapies

While we know that the immune system plays a very important role in the initiation of Long COVID symptoms, after a few months there seems to be very little utility in using medications that modulate the immune system. In the short-term, steroids seem to have some benefit in reducing the severity of the acute COVID infection, and there is some suspicion that it can reduce the likelihood of developing Long COVID. However, the risks of putting a billion people on steroids to prevent a few million cases of Long COVID makes it both difficult to study and makes the math favor not using them. In an ideal future, we will find some way of modulating the immune system after the Long COVID syndrome has developed. I will present some data on immune system drugs that have been tried in Myalgic Encephalomyelitis to help demonstrate the problem and the potential for future solutions.

Rituximab is a medication that stops the immune system from making problematic antibodies by its effect on B-Cells, which are responsible for making most of our antibodies. Of all of the medications used in rheumatology and neuroimmunology, it has one of the best safety and effectiveness profiles for many disorders, from rheumatoid arthritis to multiple sclerosis (though we use a similar type of medication called Ocrelizumab more in MS). It has been so effective that it has changed the way we think about some conditions like MS, which used to be considered a primarily T-cell mediated disorder. There was a lot of hope that rituximab would be helpful in Myalgic Encephalomyelitis, and in one small study it seemed to be useful, but in larger follow-up studies they could not find any real benefit. Because the risks are too high to start every COVID patient on a medication like Rituximab, and it does not seem to help after the post-viral syndrome has started, it is unlikely to be a very relevant treatment in Long COVID.

IL-6 Therapies

Even though it did not become a significant political hot topic like Ivermectin, hydroxychloroquine, and plasma therapy, a medication class was found to significantly help recovery in severe cases of COVID-19. Tocilizumab and similar medications block IL-6, an inflammatory cytokine that plays a significant role in organ damage during severe active COVID-19. Unfortunately, due to many factors, it was determined to only be appropriate in some of the sickest patients. The main benefit was less need for ICU treatments and improved survival rather than long-term symptom reduction. I have yet to see any analysis of these drugs affecting the development of Long COVID and most consider these treatments to have little potential for treating Long COVID.

IL-6 therapies are also used in a variety of conditions with severe neuropsychiatric symptoms, but these illnesses are fundamentally more related to delirium with an active medical cause rather than the more insidious post-viral syndrome. This syndrome is called "cytokine storm". This condition can be caused by certain other treatments of the immune system including stronger chemotherapies and a new treatment called CAR T-Cell therapies. CAR T-Cell therapies involve special immune cells that are artificially created and given to a patient to fight cancers. It is not clear to me if any long term studies have been performed on neuropsychiatric and fatigue sequelae of these medication-induced cytokine storms, but the mechanism by which they cause symptoms has many similarities to what causes the development of Long COVID after COVID-19 infection.

Other immune system drugs and Neuropsychiatric symptoms

While it has had very little supportive data, and many potential risks in the general population, a medication called hydroxychloroquine became a medical hot potato in the politico-medico-media disaster that was COVID-19. It is not entirely clear why it was ever considered as a potential treatment for the virus, but as an immune system modulator it did have some very interesting potential applications. The exact mechanism of action of hydroxychloroquine is not fully understood, but in some conditions like lupus, Sjogren's syndrome, and other rheumatologic conditions it can be quite useful. Unfortunately, its effects on the neuropsychiatric symptoms of rheumatologic diseases are extremely variable. There are many studies in "neuropsychiatric lupus" that show hydroxychloroquine can help cognitive complaints and fatigue, though the measures and definitions are arguably quite flawed. In Sjogren's syndrome, on the contrary, use of hydroxychloroquine was shown to be associated with more fatigue and other neurocognitive symptoms. Proving cause in this is nearly impossible, since hydroxychloroquine is one of the weakest disease-modifying anti-rheumatic drugs available. However, it is a very interesting potential medication to study in post-viral neurocognitive syndromes. Hopefully the extreme bias related to the medication (both bias for and bias against) will fade so it can be studied in a more reasonable fashion.

Multiple Sclerosis Therapies

Most of the immune system drugs we use in multiple sclerosis have had some data on cognitive functioning and neuropsychiatric symptoms. Interferons were one of the first classes shown to be helpful in MS, and the mood and cognitive side effects have been very well studied. They are not good. Depending on the formulation, interferons can cause symptoms that mirror severe depression and brain fog (or even severe flu-like symptoms), sometimes lasting for days after each injection. Glatiramer acetate does not have a clear neurocognitive benefit, but when compared to interferons they are less harmful. Teriflunomide (and a similar rheumatoid arthritis drug called leflunomide) have very mixed data, but seem to be at least safer, if not beneficial, in some studies on neuropsychiatric rheumatologic symptoms and psychiatric consequences of multiple sclerosis. Fingolimod (and now others like siponimod) have not been rigorously studied regarding most neurocognitive symptoms, but there was a small improvement (when compared with placebo) in a few measures of cognitive functioning in one of the landmark trials. Dimethyl fumarate (and now others like droximethyl fumarate) seem to have a good safety profile and may have some long-term protection, but, like interferons, can have flu-like or negative neurocognitive symptoms after each dose. Interestingly, one of the strongest MS disease modifying drugs called Lemtrada had some very encouraging data regarding cognitive improvement after use, but the large study that was promised (LemCog) was never fully released.

Fundamentally, while we hope to one day understand the best immune system modulating treatments, currently our data gives no clear guidance.

Some medications like interferons that reduce "inflammation in the brain" worsen depression and neurocognitive symptoms. Other treatments like teriflunomide have been shown to be good for cognition and fatigue, but only in comparison to medications that clearly worsen symptoms. Some treatments like rituximab and tocilizumab may have some benefit in preventing Long COVID, but are not safe enough to use on millions of people just to prevent the syndrome in thousands, and rituximab is not considered effective in later stages of post-infectious chronic fatigue syndrome. Some therapies like hydroxychloroquine seem to help cognition in some conditions, but hurt cognition in others.

The fundamental message is that immune system therapies may be the future of treatment, but they are not ready for regular use until better studies are performed and more data is collected. Until that time, our medications are limited to the treatment of specific symptoms of the Long COVID syndrome such as depression, insomnia, generalized fatigue, lightheadedness, migraine, and chronic pain. Even this is not some magical solution. Medications alone do not have a robust benefit in Long COVID until they are paired with other interventions described in the following chapters.

Before seeing a doctor for Long COVID, please look back at any of your previous prescriptions for the following medicines. They have all been studied for one or more symptoms in Long COVID. Note 1. when and at what dose the medicine was started, 2. what the dose was increased to, 3. if the medication had any particular effects or side effects, and 4. When and why it was stopped.

SSRIs:
Sertraline (Zoloft)
Fluoxetine (Prozac)
Citalopram (Celexa)
Escitalopram (Lexapro)
Paroxetine (Paxil)

SNRIs:
Venlafaxine (Effexor)
Desvenlafaxine (Pristiq)
Duloxetine (Cymbalta)
Milnacipran (Savella)

TCAs:
Amitriptyline (Elevil)
Nortriptyline (Pamelor)
Imipramine (Tofranil)
Doxepin (Silenor)
Clomipramine (Anafranil)

AEDs:
Levetiracetam (Keppra)

Brivaracetam (Breviact)
Topiramate (Topamax)
Zonisamide (Zonegran)
Carbamazepine (Tegretol)
Oxcarbazepine (Trileptal)
Valproate (Depakote)
Lamotrigine (Lamictal)
Gabapentin (Neurontin)

Dopamine modulating medications:
Carbidopa/Levodopa (Sinemet)
Pramipexole (Mirapex)
Ropinirole (Requip)
Rotigotine (Neupro)
Bromocriptine (Parlodel)
Cabergoline (Dostinex)
Haloperidol (Haldol)
Risperidone (Risperdal)
Chlorpromazine (Thorazine)
Olanzapine (Zyprexa)
Aripiprazole (Abilify)
Brexpiprazole (Rexulti)
Metoclopramide (Reglan)

Choline modifying medications:
Diphenhydramine (Benadryl)
Hydroxyzine (Atarax)
Scopolamine (Scop)
Trihexyphenidyl (Artane)
Benztropine (Cogentin)

Stimulants:
Methylphenidate (Ritalin/Concerta)
Amphetamine salts (Adderall, Dexedrine, Vyvanse)
Atomoxetine (Strattera)
Modafinil (Provigil)
Armodafinil (Nuvigil)
Solriamfetol (Sunosi)
Pitolisant (Wakix)

Sleep promoting medications:
Melatonin
Ramelteon (Rozerem)
Lorazepam (Ativan)
Clonazepam (Klonopin)
Diazepam (Valium)
Triazolam (Halcion)
Temazepam (Restoril)
Zaleplon (Sonata)
Zolpidem (Ambien)
Eszopiclone (Lunesta)
Suvorexant (Belsomra)
Sodium Oxybate (Xyrem)

Cardiovascular Medications:
Propranolol (Inderal)
Atenolol (Tenormin)
Metoprolol (Lopressor)
Prazosin (Minipress)
Verapamil (Verelan)

Other:

Metformin (Glucophage)
Naloxone
Naloxone/Buprenorphine (Suboxone)
Naltrexone
Ketamine

CHAPTER 6:
HOW CAN I
DO PHYSICAL
THERAPY WHEN
I CAN'T MOVE?

The most complex and contradictory literature regarding the treatment of post-infectious chronic fatigue syndrome relates to the physical approaches to treatment. In many ways, it is the conflict of allopathic medicine writ large. If you think about the body's energy as an economy, energy is taken in with breathing oxygen, eating calories, and reorganized with rest and sleep. Each muscle movement is an energy expenditure, and in Long COVID it feels that way. The treatment for exhaustion is rest. The way to cure lack of energy is to take in energy, not spend it. If it hurts when you do that, stop doing it. If it feels better when you lay down, then do that.

Intuitively, we know that all must be wrong. Surely it's not healthy to sit on a couch all day, but which physical activities or treatments are helpful in relieving symptoms, and which lead to more discomfort? Are some helpful in the long-term but painful in the moment? That feels more American, push through the pain and be rewarded for it later. No pain, no gain. Pain is weakness leaving the body. If it doesn't hurt, you're not doing it right. My patients who are driven by this childhood script start working out heavily, for about 30 minutes, and then find they can hardly move for the following 3 days, at which point they feel more fatigued and exhausted than before their spurt of motivation.

So, what is the answer then? Sit on the couch or push to exhaustion? Neither of course. The reality is there can be no blanket exercise regimen for all, and the research is complex and contradictory because no research protocol can take into account the constant troubleshooting, adjusting, and refocusing that occurs in the physical approaches to treat chronic fatigue. When we get to the 45 minute mark on our first visit, after we have discussed the problem, the different approaches to treatment, and the medications I can offer, patients invariably ask my advice about physical activity and other physical treatments. I try to speak in generalities, but they want specifics. How many minutes should they exercise? Should they do cardio or strength training? How do they deal with the fatigue when it hits? What other treatments might help them?

I cannot answer them honestly except to say that they need to decide on a physical approach to treatment and work with an expert in that discipline. Sure, as a neurologist I have learned enough to direct patients to the basics, but when it comes to troubleshooting, a good physical therapist will identify fine adjustments to make exercise more helpful, less painful, and more efficient in achieving a particular goal. The hard part is to decide which physical treatment to try, and that becomes much easier when the patient realizes there is not a right or wrong answer. I tell patients two things: "It doesn't make much sense to tell Bubba to do Yoga" and "You can't know if or how it will help until you try it." These subtle realities are hard to integrate into research, but I will try to present some of the data regarding different physical approaches to the treatment of chronic fatigue and let you decide what appeals to you.

Traditional Physical Therapy/ Occupational Therapy

In nearly all cases, the first step in treatment is to see a physical therapist and/or an occupational therapist. This is often well covered by insurance, and most doctors will be happy to write a prescription for it. While there are definitely some bad PTs out there, the vast majority of them are well-trained and have many different skills to offer. The goal is usually to assess a particular problem. First, they examine the various muscles, joints, and tissues associated with that problem. Then they come up with a treatment plan with various techniques, stretches, and exercises. Typically appointments are at least weekly, and at these appointments they will discuss progress, refine or add to the exercise regimen, and try to address barriers to improvement.

A good physical therapist will meet a patient where they are, not expecting them to do any technique that would cause excessive pain or exhaustion. They will also help patients troubleshoot barriers to success. If one type of stretching causes unwanted pain, they will watch the patient do it during the session and recommend small changes to make it more comfortable or efficient. Many physical therapists will also perform massage, needling (similar to acupuncture), electrical stimulation, cupping, and other techniques that can give both immediate relief and help reduce pain during recommended exercises for days after the appointment. Physical therapists all have various strengths and weaknesses, and one who is great at massage may not be as skilled at applying KT tape or doing electrical stimulation.

I have had many patients tell me they do not want to do physical therapy because they "tried it already". Not only were they trying it for a completely different problem, but I often find they were only doing exercises at appointments. To succeed in PT, patients have to set aside any skepticism, truly engage, have open and honest communication with the therapists about what they are doing at home, and often try a few different therapists until they find the right approach. The most common cause of failure is giving up too early, or wanting the physical therapist to do all the work. In the following sections, I write about components of physical therapy well-studied in Long COVID and similar syndromes followed by distinct physical treatment disciplines that any one physical therapist may or may not guide.

Graded Exercise Therapy

For many years, a generic term "Graded Exercise Therapy" was recommended in every guideline for the treatment of Myalgic Encephalomyelitis. In reviewing the literature, it is hard to identify exactly what is meant by graded exercise therapy other than a general concept of starting with very simple and easy exercises, stretching most importantly, and increasing slowly as patients can tolerate more and more. It is no surprise that this general guideline has led to varying results in the literature since it not only relies heavily on the patient's comfort and ability, but also the motivational skills of the therapists. More recently, there has been a spade of negative opinions regarding this therapy, with some reviews saying it is not helpful in chronic fatigue. Unfortunately, since each study has different methods, measures, and populations, the data surrounding graded exercise therapy is always going to be difficult to interpret.

However, as a concept it is very important. It is quite clear that exercise very rarely has a harmful effect long-term. It is also clear that patients with chronic fatigue, chronic pain, insomnia, migraines, dizziness, and difficulties with heart rate and shortness of breath should not start doing exercises they might have enjoyed when they were well. Too much movement clearly causes pain as well as reducing ability to function for the following day or two, leading to worsening inactivity and a punishment stimulus response. Therefore, while graded exercise therapy will always be hard to study as a "treatment", it is an obvious and necessary component of any physical approach to treatment.

The general advice is that patients should try different routines, starting very light and only increasing after they find they can tolerate it. If any specific activity (lifting, jogging, etc...) done for any particular length of time makes a patient feel like they have been hit by a bus, they must dial it back. If 40 minutes of riding an elliptical machine makes a patient feel like they are spent for the rest of the day, they should only do 30 minutes at a time until their stamina improves. Sometimes breaks help, and doing 20 minutes of exercise 3 times per day is better than 30 minutes once per day. Whether walking, jogging, stretching, lifting, or meditative breathing, patients have to discover their limits and gradually push them until they are able to tolerate more and more. For patients that have difficulty finding a good balance, a physical therapist or trainer may be able to help them structure a more accessible routine.

Cardiovascular Exercise

Cardio training is considered one of the most important types of exercise for building stamina and improving overall health, but it can be very difficult in all types of post-viral syndromes, especially Long COVID. Episodically, Long COVID patients experience a lot of sudden increases in heart rate or shortness of breath, and too much exertion can cause migraines and dizziness. Fortunately, there are other modes of exercise that can help if cardio exercises cause too much distress. It is important for patients to always remember that eventually, the ability to engage in this sort of routine is vital in recovering function. It is also good to remember that the POTS syndrome that comes with COVID is extremely variable and patients may find some days they tolerate cardio exercises even if other times they are impossible. Sometimes starting with stretches or breathing exercises can help prime the patient to then do brisk walking or other light cardio. This sort of troubleshooting can be taxing, but most patients can eventually figure out ways to add cardio to their routine slowly over time.

I try to keep my bias against running in check, but patients should be aware that the hardest cardio exercises are not the only cardio exercises. Some patients can get their heart rate and respirations quite high on stationary bikes, elliptical machines, rowing machines, or even doing dance-like stretches (pilates, martial arts, jazzercise, etc). I generally recommend patients not do anything that would cause them to travel too far until they have discovered their limits. Biking a mile away and then feeling exhausted and unable to get home can be demoralizing. It is also a good idea to find exercises you enjoy with or without a distraction like listening to music. Cardiac exercises, at their best, can also be meditative experiences if patients decide to introduce focused breathing or mental mantras.

Working with a physical therapist or physical trainer can help patients to optimize cardio exercises by working on proper posture and technique. In patients with injuries or muscle pains, slight adjustments to how a patient walks can truly become life saving. This can be a slow process with frequent adjustments as one technique may change which muscle groups are over taxed and need to be further modified. This can be a fun process or a frustrating one depending on the patient and the therapist, but when someone can really start increasing their stamina it can have amazing benefits for fatigue as well as other body systems affected in Long COVID. However, it is important to remember that while most people can safely do a good cardiac regimen, close monitoring by your primary care doctor is vital in case of chest pain or new types of shortness of breath. While very rare, COVID-19 can cause other medical conditions such as heart and lung inflammation and blood clotting problems.

Strength Training

As previously discussed, COVID-19, post-acute COVID, and Long COVID can involve a very unfortunate feedback loop whereby pain and weakness lead to inactivity leading to further pain and weakness. Many patients seen in the neurology office have a lot of muscle atrophy, especially in the upper arms and thighs. These patients cannot do any cardio exercise at all because they are fundamentally too weak from decompensation. In these cases, strength training is a very important and early intervention to help them tolerate the other forms of physical activity. This often requires close monitoring with a physical trainer or physical therapist because strengthening muscle groups needs to be done in a planned and rational way. Also, strengthening the upper legs and pelvic muscles often requires balancing in various ways that can be unsafe and lead to falls if not guided by a professional. Often there will be a list of exercises done at home, and a list of exercises that require assistance.

Strength training and posture are also very important for cognitive functioning. We do not fully understand all of the mechanisms, but strengthening the lower extremity extensors (the leg muscles required to stand from a crouched position) seems to have a unique effect on positive outlook, overall metabolism, and energy level. Core strengthening (abdomen and back musculature) is also very important for stabilizing respirations, heart rate, and other organ function. Strengthening and stretching the pelvic floor and hip muscles is closely connected with both intestinal and urinary health as well as sexual functioning. We know that posture and strength in all of these muscle groups are a major part of how more complex techniques like yoga and Tai Chi help, though the exact connection between strengthening and neurocognitive symptoms has not been thoroughly studied. Fundamentally, basic strengthening is required for patients to be able to tolerate other techniques like yoga and Tai Chi, which have the most data surrounding their efficacy in post-viral chronic fatigue syndromes like Myalgic Encephalomyelitis and Long COVID.

Yoga/Stretching Techniques

Likely due to its popular appeal, yoga has been the most well-studied physical modality in Myalgic Encephalomyelitis and Long COVID. Unfortunately, because it is a complex process, the literature is very difficult to navigate from a medical science perspective. Yoga's long history has involved a waxing and waning narrative between a mental and spiritual practice and a physical one. At its best it is an integration of both, but there are many who believe that the core mental and spiritual practice is too enmeshed with Eastern philosophy to properly translate into the Western world. Some yogic practices are difficult to even describe in English, and books could be written just on the topic of how the Western world has misinterpreted yogic Eastern philosophy. There is no point in belaboring this except to say that all of the literature on yoga as a medical treatment should be understood as limited by nature. Whatever this thing is that has been filtered through Western culture seems to have some usefulness in treatment.

One study out of Japan evaluating yoga showed not only improvements in fatigue and energy, but also found reduced cortisol and TNF-a. The same study showed improvements in shortness of breath and heart rate stability as well as heart rate variability, considered a possible marker for overall cardiac and autonomic health. However, most of the data is mixed. One study will show statistically significant improvements in fatigue, pain, depression, or insomnia while another will not. The biggest criticism in review articles relates to the low number of patients and the potential for bias, but there is no data to suggest it is harmful, and the nature of yoga makes it particularly interesting in Long COVID. The core feature of yoga is that it is a modality of combining strength, flexibility, and balance with relaxation, mindfulness, and breath work. This integration of different components that are all part of the post-viral syndrome make it highly likely to have some benefits. Like all other physical therapies, however, it is also dependent upon the patient, practitioner, and setting. Generally, finding a yogic practice and guide who match the perspective of the patient is key. Trying to get a spiritual person to do yoga in a purely mechanical model, or a very non-spiritual person to do yoga in a religious model, will likely be ineffective.

Tai Chi/Qigong

Similar to yoga, Tai Chi and other disciplines like Qigong have been studied in all manner of Long Covid symptoms, though there is very limited research yet on Long Covid patients. Tai Chi and Qigong are both meditative movement practices that are also extremely variable in the West. They typically involve specific choreographed movements that are slow and intentional, like a well-honed dance, as well as intensive meditation with specific structural disciplines focusing on parts of the body acting as houses for emotional energy. Translating this metaphor into allopathic medicine is likely not ever going to be compatible. However, if we abandon the metaphysics of Tai Chi, it is a much more regimented practice, making research into its use for neurologic conditions more consistent.

A recent analysis not only showed improvements in overall health measures, but also improved brain network functioning. While functional MRI has had plenty of criticism, the most current model that looks at network dysfunction showed that when Tai Chi improved quality of life measures (specifically pain), it also improved brain network functioning. Interestingly, it gives further credence to the overlap between the pain and depression networks in the brain since reported decreases in pain were closely correlated with network improvement in the areas most well-known to be involved with depression. Tai Chi (and Qigong) have been studied as effective treatments for similar symptoms that can also be present in Parkinson's and multiple sclerosis.

One of the main benefits of Tai Chi and Qigong are that they do not require significant flexibility and balance, often needed for even "moderate" yoga poses. This means they can be started and practiced consistently in patients who are still struggling with generalized weakness and balance difficulties, though dizziness and migraine are often still limiting factors.

Acupuncture/Cupping/Moxibustion

While some patients get anxious when I begin to discuss acupuncture with them, a surprising number of patients tell me they have been thinking about it. They will have heard about its benefits with pain, but they rarely have an idea of how diverse and effective the treatments can be for a whole host of Long COVID symptoms. Acupuncture is one of many disciplines within Traditional Chinese Medicine (TCM) as well as traditional medicine practices of many cultures in the near and far East. Other physical disciplines include moxibustion, massage, and cupping. While the Chinese will rightfully say they have thousands of years of data on how TCM treatments work, Western medicine has been very skeptical of this. Though modern medicine has tested acupuncture quite well for a variety of symptoms and the data is reassuring, Chinese medical philosophy has always been difficult to integrate in any way with Western medical philosophy. A Chinese medical provider may feel your pulses (technically 3 pulses on each arm at 3 depths), look at your tongue, and diagnose a patient with wind in their liver, a deficiency of Yin. Acupuncture points will be chosen based on their map of meridians to unblock the flow of Qi that happens in this condition. This language has no direct correlate in Western medicine, so no matter the treatments' efficacy, there has always been a hard wall between the two medical worlds.

I will not try to explain what I have learned about acupuncture and similar treatments, but will leave that to the trained TCM practitioner. However, the past twenty years has seen an explosion of literature into the physiologic processes happening from a Western perspective during acupuncture treatment.

Some dismiss these studies as a study of the "placebo method", but that does not account for the robust data regarding both efficacy and changes to brain activity when comparing active treatment to "sham treatments", which should have a similar effect if it were all placebo. The most interesting data from a neuropsychiatric perspective is the change to functional brain activity during acupuncture of specific acupoints, as well as biomarker data in hormone disorders like hypothyroidism. It is important not to focus on the Western analysis and think we understand acupuncture, since the Eastern model is still required to form a treatment plan and thus has superiority to Western medicine with regards to conceptualizing its effects.

In Long COVID patients, only small trials or case reports have been published, but in migraine, fatigue, pain, insomnia, mood disorders, and other components of the Long COVID syndrome the research is robust. Each study is limited by some factor or another, but the majority of them show efficacy well above some medications. The main problem is the integration of Western and Eastern approaches, so the patients may all have the same Western diagnosis (primary insomnia) but they might have a variety of TCM diagnoses. This gets more complex when trying to compare TCM with acupuncture traditions from other countries and disciplines. This is too much for a Western doctor to be expected to learn about, and yet acupuncture referrals have become nearly mainstream with patients expressing significant improvement in symptoms. One absolute superiority is the ability to get acupuncture treatments despite muscle pain and fatigue that might still limit exercise, though needle phobia and potential for unexpected mood and sleep changes can occur.

Massage/Structural Integration

Though it has a much longer tradition in Western medicine, massage and other disciplines of physical soft tissue manipulation are not necessarily better understood. It makes sense to us (more than inserting and twisting needles) that massaging a muscle should make it feel better, but the complex autonomic and vagal neurologic response to different types of touch is extremely complex. Even light touch or simulated touch can have major effects on the nervous system. Emotional touch, such as holding, plays a major role in addition to the relaxation of the muscles from deep massage. There has been an attempt to integrate Western medical science and anatomy with massage, more so than with acupuncture, with discussions of lymphatic drainage, blood vessel changes and growth, and fluid dynamics, but these are very hard to integrate into a practice, and have never truly shaped the fields of massage therapy with regard to technique.

Furthermore, like with acupuncture, there are many

different disciplines of massage that might have different physiologic effects on the body. Some might include "energy-work" like Reiki or massage that integrates yoga techniques, while others have a full structural perspective with the goal of realigning the body. The core philosophy of any one massage discipline or any one practitioner may have unique components that they have found helpful for clients. I tend to recommend patients give any individual therapist at least 3-4 sessions to determine if they are getting improvement, and then to switch to a different modality. Unfortunately, each modality might have different schools that make them distinct. However, I have learned not to try to predict which modality will have the greatest impact on an individual's symptoms.

Chiropractic Treatments

Of all of the physical approaches, chiropractic medicine has always been a fascinating contradiction. It has garnered more acceptance as a medical art in the West than any other physical approach, but the philosophical mindset and apparent differences between providers puts it far outside the Western approach to medical science. Do not imagine this is a criticism, but simply an observation. Physical therapists will use Traditional Chinese Medicine techniques and as far as I can tell, they completely divorce the technique from traditional Chinese philosophy. This bothers me much more deeply because it is a stolen art used with completely fabricated justifications. Physical therapists do "dry needling" that resembles acupuncture, use the Eastern acupuncture literature to justify their needle placements, but they remove all concepts of meridian lines, energies, and vessels out of hand. It would be like a physical therapist recommending aspirin to prevent stroke, but not considering any of the Western scientific theories of how aspirin works, instead making something up like "aspirin irritates the stomach leading to realignment of the fascia which reshapes the bloodvessel."

Chiropractic medicine holds true to its origins, in many ways, which I deeply respect. I also know that it works because of how my patients respond to it. However, it seems more like magic to me than acupuncture or even prayer or energy work, which have more obvious brain networks modulating them. For a chiropractor to say that popping a certain joint in a certain way can relieve sinus congestion due to allergies baffles me, but my patients' experience of it working is sufficient for me to tell them to keep doing it.

There are so many historical influences on chiropractic treatments that they probably cannot be summarized in any one resource. A huge influence comes from the older Western medical discipline of Osteopathic medicine. Modern Osteopaths (given the title of D.O.) are trained so similar to M.D.s that they are nearly impossible to differentiate. They may have a small amount of coursework on massage or joint and tissue manipulation, but as recently as 50 years ago they were a completely different discipline with an almost opposite philosophy. The allopathic physician (M.D.) saw human illness as either a deficiency or an excess of a natural process, and their job was to do the opposite (allo means other/opposite). Thyroid too low? Add thyroid hormone. Thyroid too high? Lets remove some thyroid or block it. The osteopathic philosophy was simply that the body was capable of healing, but illness came because the body was not properly aligned. If you align the body, the body will do the rest. Chiropractic medicine definitely uses this core philosophy, which could explain how an alignment could fix nearly any medical problem. However, I am still skeptical of the logical connections they use to explain their results.

Physical Therapies In Long Covid

In truth, this is one of the most vital components of treatment in Long COVID, but the one that I am least able to motivate patients to engage with. It costs patients more to see a good massage therapist than their co-pays to see me three times in the neurology clinic and pick up the medication I prescribe. It is also a big time investment, with even standard PT being at least weekly (usually twice weekly) for 8-12 weeks. Even if they cannot understand all of the ways psychotherapy can help, insurance often pays and at worst they can justify that they are paying for an hour of friendship that costs much less than a dinner date.

With acupuncture, patients cannot quite get how or why it would help, they often have to pay out of pocket, and that is before the needle phobia kicks in. Fortunately, I have found that patients are pretty responsive to the recommendation, showing interest in my thoughts and describing how they have always wanted to give it a try. Unfortunately, patients will often never make a phone call or will give up after the first session if they do not see immediate results, and they never tell me they gave up on it unless I press them.

There is another big problem for some patients, especially those who want to be told what to do rather than to be given information and options. For me, figuring out which therapy and which therapist or even which modality of therapy will help a patient the most is nearly impossible. However, with well designed naturalistic studies, all of these physical therapies have been shown to have great benefits for nearly all of the symptoms in Long COVID. Some, like acupuncture, yoga, and Tai Chi have been found to have fascinating effects on the immune system markers that go awry in post-viral syndromes like Long COVID. These may be completely different mechanisms, or they may be related, but there is no surprise that my Long COVID patients have responded well when they have done these therapies in conjunction with medical treatments, psychotherapy, and other therapeutics.

When patients are at a loss of which to try first, I give the same advice. If the patient feels they would enjoy one more, or would be more hopeful about a specific technique, I tell them to go with that one. It is far easier to stay motivated with a chiropractor when you have friends who have benefited in the past or had a positive personal experience before with that mode of treatment. If a patient "believes" in a certain modality, then I am far more likely to recommend it than if they start from a place of skepticism. I definitely do not think that acupuncture is "all placebo" since I have been involved in research showing the changes in the brain that modulate its effects, but if it ALSO has a placebo effect, all the better. Moreover, if a patient is too skeptical they can have a "Nocebo" effect, where an otherwise effective treatment does not work due to the patient's low expectations. This even works with medicines. There are studies showing that if you give someone a strong opiate, and tell them it is "just a tylenol", it does not work nearly as well as if they are not told what it is.

I also tell patients to stay hopeful for at least 3-4 sessions with any practitioner. Often the first few sessions they are getting to know the patient and slowly adjusting their technique. After the 4th session, if a patient is really expecting it to fail, I also recommend they discuss this with the therapist. While open communication about these issues can be very hard for patients, the results of that discussion can be very helpful. In some cases, the therapist will change their approach, and in other cases the therapist will agree that it is not working and recommend a colleague who might be better in the patient's particular case. At that point, the therapist knows a lot more about the patient's history, body, and problem than anyone else and they often know most of the other local therapists. This makes them an extremely valuable referral source.

In the end, I am happier for a patient to do online beginners yoga and go on daily walks (graded exercise fashion) than to feel too overwhelmed by picking between acupuncture and chiropractic medicine. I have found some patients really like having options, while others want a lot of benevolent paternalistic direction. In the end, though, if I see a patient once every three months as their neurologist, and all of their motivation comes from my 30 minute discussion with them, then they will not start a good routine until 9-12 months in. By then, half of the work will be treating their muscle atrophy and cardio-respiratory decompensation. It is much easier to start doing any physical therapy 3 months into Long COVID than a year into it.

If you or a loved one is really struggling, the best thing to do is get started. If you are skeptical, try to simply suspend the disbelief. I have learned a lot about this from the folks in recovery with AA. Accept that you are powerless over your fatigue and that your weakness has become unmanageable. You need a higher power (like this book) to overcome it. Take a clear and honest inventory of your daily exercise and how much time you spend on the couch reading social media posts and watching cat videos. You can skip the apologies, but you should honestly admit to yourself and one other person how hard it can be to start exercising. And then find a program and go to meetings. It works if you work it, so work it, you are worth it. Now go out there and get your body moving. A body at rest wants to stay at rest, but your body needs to start moving, so put down this book now and go on a short walk.

CHAPTER 7: HOW IS TALKING GOING TO HELP?

In Chapter 1, I discussed that the main difference I see between Neurology and Psychiatry is stigma. The causes for this broadly sweeping societal prejudice are beyond the scope of this book, but it must be addressed because there is a lot of resistance to seeking psychotherapeutic help in conditions like Long COVID. When some doctors recommend psychotherapy, patients often respond by thinking "So you think it's all in my head?" or "So you think I'm crazy?". However, it is recommended because psychotherapy can be immensely helpful for patients and families struggling with Long COVID. Psychotherapy is at its heart focused on facilitating human change. Helping individuals better adjust to and cope with the myriad changes they face throughout their lifespan is an essential component of all good psychotherapeutic approaches. Working with a good therapist can have an enormous positive impact on symptom severity, healing and recovery, and creating a path forward through and beyond this terrible illness.

Psychotherapy has had a complex history within the academic medical literature. While neurologists were shocking people's muscles and dog's brains to determine the structure of the nervous system, other health professionals were finding that a basic conversational approach could also modify the brain. It sounds easy, but some patients feel sharing their most private thoughts with another human is more invasive than a lobotomy. These early approaches were flawed and raw, but "the talking cure" clearly improved patients' functioning and quality of life, and behaviorists showed that simple techniques could reinforce or extinguish target behaviors that have a huge impact on other health measures. Modern psychology has discovered new avenues by which to treat these brain network problems, typically focused on syndromes like anxiety and depression. What therapists may or may not know is that their techniques to modify the brain do not just control mood related symptoms, but can have a dramatic impact on every other system of the body with only minor modifications to their techniques.

I am admittedly biased, believing the brain is the core driver of the other systems in the human body. Intellectually, I can accept that the liver can have an equally powerful effect on the brain, but I just cannot shake the view that the brain is a more useful place to intervene. Sure, I can give someone lactulose and wake liver failure patients from a coma, but I can prevent liver failure most of the time by getting someone into a good substance use disorder rehab program. I know we can keep the brain alive with a heart transplant, but through modifying behavior (diet, exercise) and mood with meditation and psychotherapy, we might save them from the need for such an invasive and temporizing procedure. Patients are able to diet and exercise without psychotherapy. However, the addition of both behavioral and psychological techniques can make dieting and exercise much easier, as well as reduce inflammation and hormone imbalances caused by stress.

Unfortunately, psychotherapeutic techniques can be much more complex and difficult to analyze in research studies than pills or surgical procedures. In most cases, psychotherapeutic techniques are profoundly and obviously effective to anyone in patient care, but the trial data is often less clear. Subtle differences in populations, difficulty measuring mood and behavior changes, and the challenge of reducing a disorder like depression or anxiety down to numbers on a page make research very difficult. Consequently, good research into psychotherapy for Long COVID (and Myalgic Encephalomyelitis before it) has been limited by what is measurable and what can be analyzed. One of the most famous early minds in modern American industry, W. Edwards Demming, has two quotes that summarize this struggle: "Trust in God [if you must], but everyone else must bring data." and "The most important things to consider often cannot be measured." Despite this difficulty, nearly all providers will agree that psychotherapy is vital in the treatment of Long COVID symptoms.

Resistance

Many people reading this book have been in therapy in the past, and for many of them it did not go well. I consider these folks vaccinated against therapy: just enough of it to build up a resistance. Maybe you know therapy could help with problems you have had for ages, but never got treatment because you could push through without it. Now you have Long COVID. Now your symptoms make it hard or even impossible to complete vital tasks. Your doctors tell you that talking to someone for an hour a week will go a long way to helping you feel better, but you do not understand because this is not just anxiety. This is a real medical illness. Seems like a tall order, right? My hope is that this chapter will walk you through various aspects of the process by which you can evaluate if and how psychotherapy can help, to identify the modality or "type" of therapy that might be the best fit for your personal preferences, and to determine for yourself whether a particular therapist will be helpful in the short-term, or if they would help for the long haul.

Which type of psychotherapy is right for you? This is a difficult question, and it does not have a straightforward answer. What the literature has clearly shown is that the answers are not clear at all. One study will show a particular psychotherapy is very effective, if not vital, for the treatment of a disorder. A second study will show it has little benefit beyond basic education. Is this researcher bias? Perhaps, but now the research has clearly shown there are a few important factors that make a psychotherapy effective or ineffective, and it has nothing to do with the choice between the various cognitive, behavioral, and psychodynamic approaches.

The core question patients ask me is not should I do DBT, EMDR, or IFS. They ask "Why would talking about my day help my leg pain?" They say, "I did therapy before and it was worthless." They ask, "What if I spend all my time telling someone all about me, and they aren't any good?" Patients will explain to me why therapy could harm them, but they are curious to try a drug that takes a sledgehammer to the immune system. Patients are often more willing to spend $800/month on a pill that helped a friend of theirs with a different problem than take a risk on therapy. So I negotiate with them. I say to give a therapist 4 sessions, see if they feel the therapist is listening, seems to share an understanding of their goals, and seems to care. I also say that if they do not think it is working out they should go to one more session and tell the therapist what they are feeling and see if they think a different therapist might be better for them.

What I rarely divulge is that I am telling them to keep an eye out for the most important components of good therapy, the common factors.

Common Factors

The common factors for effective therapy rely on a combination of the therapist's personality and training and the patient's personality and perspectives. Simply speaking, while the development of common factors are impossible to predict, they can be easily recognized and fostered by the therapist. It is not a patient's responsibility to know or focus on these, but I do think it is reasonable for a patient to find a new therapist if they are clearly not present. The most well-studied common factors are 1. a good therapeutic alliance, 2. the therapist's empathy as perceived by the patient, 3. a sense of unconditional positive regard, 4. how genuine the therapist is or seems, and 5. reasonable client expectations.

Generally, the patient and the therapist must have an agreement on some level that a particular approach should be used for a particular goal. If the patient wants to stop having panic attacks or to get more comfortable being in public, and the therapist wants the patient to become enlightened by talking about how they hate their mother, it probably will not be an effective treatment. Much of this negotiation happens by reading the context rather than a formal therapy plan, and it should be flexible as new material arises. However, some therapists are inflexible and some patients have an unreasonable expectation that the therapist can fix thirty years of maladaptive behavioral patterns without any discomfort on the patient's part.

For any therapy course to be useful, a therapist must develop some empathy and positive regard towards the patient that the patient can sense or believe. The therapist should not get drawn into the patient's misery, but they should be able to sense it and have a feeling in response to it. The therapist may even hate what a patient is doing, but that hate should be toward the behavior, and perhaps for the negative impacts of that behavior on the patient's life, not the patient as a person. Toward patients themselves, a therapist should convey a sense of warmth, acceptance, support, and respect. If any of these things are lacking, or if the therapist feels defensive to you when you try to discuss any of these factors, it might not be the best fit.

While most of the common factors are related to general compatibility, shared goals, shared perspectives, and responsiveness to each other, there are some core responsibilities of both parties. The therapist cannot rely on mechanical empathy, or truly hide feelings of discomfort. Genuineness is a core feature, and if a therapist is just trying to pretend they care, the therapy will not be very effective. The patient must be honest about their expectations and feelings, and they must accept that some goals are more achievable than others, or that some goals must be achieved before others will be possible.

The real secret is that these common features are just as important in cardiology as they are in psychology. We all know this instinctively. Doctors are taught the absolute basics of this in their medical training: lean forward, smile, remember the patient is suffering. Doctors are even asked to answer multiple choice questions about how to respond to patients who are suffering. Beyond that, there is little education about humanism and empathy in structured medical training.

So now that you know a little about what psychotherapy is, the common factors that make it function, and feel you might, just maybe, be willing to give it a go, what next? The process of getting in with a therapist who feels safe, empathic, accepts your insurance, and is a good fit can be overwhelming. If you call the number on the back of your insurance card, they will email or fax you a seemingly endless list of options that may or may not be out of date. Alternatively, you might live in a part of the country where there are only three options on that list and they all know you socially. Once you finally find websites for providers who seem competent, friendly enough, and take your insurance, their websites might be full of jargon. Acronyms like CBT, DBT, ACT, REBT, ABA, etc often precede proud declarations that this or that method is the current, evidence-based gold standard treatment. How is a patient to tell which therapy would help them?

Below is a brief introduction to several of the most common, and a few less common, methods of psychotherapy available today. I include some of the philosophy of each followed by my impression of why one might be particularly helpful for certain patients. These are only cursory descriptions. Each method of therapy outlined below has been written about and studied *ad nauseum*. Each has tomes written about its theory and practice, but we cannot expect patients to become a scholar on the topic before they pick a type of therapy.

Person-Centered Psychotherapy

Also sometimes referred to as humanistic or Rogerian psychotherapy, this approach re-entered the landscape with the help of Carl Rogers. He believed we have an idealized version of ourselves that often differs substantially from our daily reality. Rogers believed human suffering was caused, in part, by the impossibility of reconciling the realities of our lives with the idealized, aspirational fantasies we construct of who we would like to be. He also felt that individuals have a deep, internal understanding of themselves and the nature of their sufferings, and an internal drive to bridge the gap between their current and idealized selves.

Because of this internal drive toward healing and

wholeness, which he called a self-actualizing urge, Rogers advised a non-directive approach with a heavy emphasis on the common factors. Current Rogerian, humanistic, or person-centered clinicians strive to embody the warmth, genuineness, accurate empathy and understanding outlined in the common factors. They believe by meeting patients wherever they are on a given day and helping them explore their experiences, individuals will naturally talk their way toward what is most central to their current distress and future healing. This usually involves reconciling who you would like to be with the realities of your current situation, limitations, and struggles along the way.

So you are tired, so tired, and the drudgery of pressing on through these exhausting symptoms has left you feeling low and disconnected from the industrious worker you were once so proud to be. You question whether you are the person everyone thinks you are. Maybe they always had an unrealistic idea of your potential, capacity, and contribution. Worse, maybe you now worry you have always secretly been this tired, lazy, or weak. A person-centered therapist would begin by getting a sense of who you are, what matters to you, and how you are doing right now. This type of clinician will let you direct the session, largely, but will occasionally offer observations, reflections, or feedback. Sessions will likely feel somewhat like conversations with a very supportive friend, who happens to ask the right questions to guide you suddenly to revealing your own solutions.

Individuals struggling with Long COVID symptoms often question their sense of self-worth, self-esteem, or identity. Some of them will prefer supportive listening and the freedom to talk through their experiences at their own direction. These patients would likely find supportive person-centered therapeutic approaches especially helpful. It may also be a necessary first step before transitioning to more complex treatments. Like learning to swim, it would be dangerous to dive into deep waters without feeling safe near the surface.

Supportive Psychotherapy

Supportive therapy is an informal term often used by providers to describe a psychotherapy relationship in which the primary interventions are supportive listening and gentle exploration of a patient's experience of their life and struggles from week to week. This bears a lot of resemblance to the Rogerian, person-centered approach in its warmth and attunement. Although some describe supportive therapists as "friends for hire" and criticize its relatively loose structure, common factors research and conventional clinical wisdom both indicate that relationships, not treatment methods, help people heal and affect personal change. For individuals struggling with Long COVID symptoms, supportive therapy can be a safe place to dedicate to self care each week. It can be a place to discuss their daily highs and lows, and collaboratively strategize ways to navigate Long COVID symptoms and their impact on work and life.

Maybe getting through the day with your Long COVID symptoms is manageable, however depleting, and you feel you might benefit from a "sounding board". Perhaps regular sessions of talking out your difficulties, strategizing practical solutions, and generally exploring various aspects of your life could be just what you need. With a supportive psychotherapist, weekly or bi-weekly therapy can help many patients manage the social, professional/ academic, financial, and survival needs required for continued living with Long COVID.

Cognitive Behavioral Therapy

Cognitive Behavioral Therapy (CBT) is often touted as the "gold standard" treatment modality of the modern era. CBT operates on the assumption that our thoughts, behaviors, and emotional experiences are interconnected. How we feel is directly influenced by what we think and what we do. Think for a moment about your happiest memory. Really put yourself back there. See if you can imagine it so vividly you can almost smell and feel the various facets of the memory. Set a timer for 30 seconds and continue to sit, eyes closed in this memory. When the timer sounds, stop.

How did you feel? My guess is that your feelings and the sensations in your body had a similar tone to the contents of the memory. Now imagine that as we go through the day, every thought we generate has the potential to create a tiny little version of an emotion. Think of the number of thoughts you had the last time you were running late for an important engagement. Picture what thoughts come up automatically at every yellow light. Imagine the frustrations that accompany those thoughts.

CBT utilizes structured session formats, therapeutic "homework", and often psychometric questionnaires to establish baselines and monitor progress to shape those thoughts, feelings, and behaviors into a more helpful dynamic. In order to meet those goals, a CBT therapist will work with you to gain insight into your thoughts, the behaviors you engage in, and the ways both impact your emotional life and decision making. There are well-validated CBT protocols tailored to a variety of symptoms and syndromes including anxiety and depression as well as fatigue and chronic pain.

CBT might be a great fit for clients whose experience of Long COVID has led to the development of one or two easily identifiable symptoms they would like to reduce or eliminate via a structured, goal-directed method. For example, if Long COVID symptoms such as fatigue and brain fog have worn you down, or the anxiety related to loss of productivity is overwhelming, you may benefit from a short course of CBT treatment.

Acceptance And Commitment Therapy

Acceptance and Commitment Therapy (ACT) is another fairly structured, evidence-supported treatment modality. ACT is considered an experiential and behavioral method and includes some of the structured components characteristic of CBT (e.g. homework assignments or mindfulness practices). It also emphasizes, without judgment, the role we often play in perpetuating our own distress. Like CBT, ACT posits that our life is heavily impacted by what we think, say, and do. Unlike CBT, ACT posits that most suffering can be traced back to language and a sense of being inappropriately fused with our thoughts, the way we turn them into language, and the ways we perpetuate our own miseries through our behaviors.

The ACT approach utilizes metaphors, directed mindfulness, and exercises to help patients understand their distress. It helps patients gain insight into how the things they have previously tried to solve their problems have been unhelpful. Through this, patients develop willingness to try things in new ways. Patients can then experiment to find new, more adaptive ways to navigate their lives and struggles.

ACT might be especially helpful for those Long COVID patients who find themselves "stuck in their heads" or for individuals who "learn by doing". It is also a good fit for folks who need concrete data as a way to track progress. ACT is also firmly grounded in individuals' personal values. Those who are unaware of or disconnected from their values can find ACT especially helpful. Once they gain insight/awareness into their values and begin making values-congruent behavioral changes to decrease their psychic distress, symptom reduction and habit changes are much easier.

Dialectic Behavioral Therapy

DBT is a comprehensive, cognitive behavioral approach to therapy with a vast body of research literature supporting its efficacy for different clinical populations and presentations. It utilizes five modules (mindfulness, distress tolerance, interpersonal effectiveness, emotion regulation, and "walking the middle path"). Each of those modules can be used to teach ideas, skills, and techniques used to make psychological distress more manageable. A key tenet of this approach is that "You may not have caused your problems, and they are not your fault, but only you have the power to fix them." There is a real tough-love component to DBT and a fundamental emphasis on personal responsibility. Patients dealing with issues related to Long COVID who value a high degree of structure and enjoy having concrete, easily referenced "how-to" guides often do especially well in

DBT.

DBT also conceptualizes most facets of therapy as skill building, which can make it feel a little like you are learning to play a new game rather than lying on a couch contemplating your childhood. The interpersonal effectiveness skills might be especially noteworthy for Long COVID patients. You know you used to be able to do so much more, and you feel like those around you expect you to perform like you used to. Maybe now you feel embarrassed or ashamed or like you just "can't cut it". You have no clue how to explain this to those around you. They may look to you for support, task completion, or advice, and right now you just cannot do it. An entire module of DBT centers around the development of structured, repeatable skills for self-advocacy, conflict resolution, and interpersonal disagreement. Mindfulness can be used to manage the experience of certain symptoms, distress tolerance, and emotion regulation. This can be extremely helpful for getting through the terrible physical symptoms of Long COVID. "Walking the middle path" can be helpful toward accepting your current limitations and learning to find joy as you progress on your journey. If any of this resonates with your experiences, DBT may be a good choice to speed your recovery.

Internal Family Systems Therapy

Maybe you are not like any of the Long COVID

patients I have discussed so far. Maybe a part of you is doing "just fine". Maybe a part of you gets tired at the end of the day, sure, but who doesn't? Maybe part of you feels like a helpless child in the mornings when you wake and face your day, but we all do, right? Compartmentalization is a part of life. We all do it, but since COVID you have had a harder time compartmentalizing to get through the day than you used to. If you could just leave behind that tired part of you that feels overwhelmed, you know you would be fine. Maybe a little extra compartmentalization could help you out, but it could be that Long COVID is revealing you were not quite so thoroughly compartmentalized as you had thought.

IFS is rooted in the idea that we all have different "parts" of ourselves. There is a part of you that wants to lose weight, perhaps, which is distinctly different from the part of you that craves an ice cream sundae every night. IFS posits that we experience psychological distress when these parts become unbalanced.

In terms of Long COVID, part of you could have made a degree of peace with your current situation even as another part of you feels hopeless about the future. Maybe you feel like your adjustment to living with the symptoms of Long COVID is a bit disjointed or fragmented. Perhaps you feel as though your thoughts, feelings, or beliefs about your Long COVID symptoms, yourself, and your future seem to change on a dime. If so, IFS clinicians might be a good fit to help you sort through these conflicted feelings. With IFS, you can gain insight into the different "parts of yourself" that have likely been playing an influential role in your daily internal life. Of note, this method tends to be fairly relational in execution, and strong emotional experiences often occur in the clinical encounters. People can get pretty angry at the parts of themselves that are not helping them achieve their goals. Healing can be dramatic when patients begin to have some compassion for these parts of themselves.

Depth Psychodynamic Approaches

Depth-oriented dynamic approaches are numerous and vary in their methods of intervention and timeline. Some depth-oriented dynamic approaches are designed to be implemented in relatively few sessions (6-20) and some utilize hundreds of sessions over spans of many years. Their common denominators tend to be the illumination of the unconscious and a focus on "defenses", as well as an idea that our formative years and early experiences have an impact on how we develop and who we become later in life. We all utilize defense mechanisms in our daily lives such as suppressing anger when a boss gives you upsetting news. Unfortunately, when these defenses are employed without our knowledge or intention, they can start to drive our lives where we do not want to go. Suppressing anger at work might prove so effective so often that we begin suppressing all "negative emotions" until eventually we feel disconnected from ourselves and our loved ones.

In terms of Long COVID, the symptoms themselves often necessitate the development of new adaptive coping strategies with new, more effective defenses. In the process of adjusting to major life changes, new struggles may be guided by how we previously navigated other difficult emotional challenges. Depth-oriented dynamic approaches will help you explore who you are and how you came to be this way, discern who you would like to be moving forward, become more aware of your defenses, and improve your ability to intentionally choose when and how you react to different stressors. These are the approaches that tend to emphasize early life, talking about your childhood, and reflecting deeply on the influences that led to your current situation. If you would rather never talk about how you are still angry at your mother and how this has led you to hate who you are with Long COVID, one of the previous approaches may be more appropriate for you.

Existential Therapies

Existential therapies are characterized by a belief that there are certain key experiences of being alive that are universal to all people. We all have experiences of loneliness, death, freedom of will, etc. Our inevitable deaths lend a sense of urgency and meaning to our lives. Existential providers will conceptualize issues as they relate to these core anxieties and our overall process of "meaning-making" about our lives and identities. What do these Long COVID symptoms you are contending with now mean for your sense of personal autonomy? What do they mean for the rest of your life? Who are you, really, in relationship to others? Have you always been defined by your work?

Existential approaches to psychotherapy may have particular value if you are struggling with "the big questions". Our culture often dismisses these issues leading patients to feel alone in their struggles. The world is a mess, and every article on Facebook leads to further despair. However, addressing those existential issues can reshape nearly everything about a person's perspective. If Long COVID has left you doubting your self worth, or the value of life in general, or if you are dealing with a major loss or questions about your own mortality, an existential psychotherapist may be particularly helpful.

Formal Psychoanalysis

If you are interested in a deep dive into your history, the complexes that shape your personality, and the connection between your early development, drives, and behaviors, there are some practitioners who still provide psychoanalysis. Because this process is very long and time/labor intensive, it is rarely covered by insurance. While some modern psychologists and psychiatrists dismiss psychoanalysis as impractical, those who provide this service would consider it to be the ultimate treatment modality for the psyche. Other psychotherapies can modify behaviors, reduce symptoms, and improve emotions, but only psychoanalysis examines the nature of the self, and why our unique experiences in childhood and daily life shape how we feel and behave.

These practitioners may utilize dream analysis, free association, or transference to help softly guide a patient towards a better understanding of their core nature. Most practitioners are either Freudian or Neofreudian, examining the most innate drives and discovering how suppression of these drives leads to maladaptive coping strategies, all much deeper than the conscious brain processes. Other modalities may more quickly result in symptom reduction and effective habit changes, but if you want to understand who you are and who you could be on the deepest level, psychoanalysis could be the best treatment for you.

Analytical Psychology

A student of Freud, Carl Jung, developed a correlate of Freudian psychoanalysis that differs in some core ways from the classical approach. Rather than a chaotic unconscious mostly filled with animalistic drives relating to sexual urges, Jung and his students examined the structure of the psyche, the persona, the complexes, the transcendental function, the Archetypes, and ultimately the Self. While some Jungian schools are criticized as being more religious than psychological, that is reductionistic, treating their metaphors as equivalent to the myths that they were drawn from.

The classical school of analytical psychology helps patients to gradually discover which stories and myths are manifesting in their lives, where these motifs originate, and begin to integrate with the deepest component of the psyche: the Self. If you have been having deeply disturbing experiences that resemble stories from classical literature, feel your unconscious trying to "speak to you" through dreams, or otherwise feel that knowing yourself is more important than fixing any individual problem, analytical psychology may be appropriate for you. Freud classically said the purpose of his method was to enable patients to work and love effectively. If you want to retire and let go, Jung's approach may be helpful.

Too Much?

After starting therapy, many of my patients describe a concern that they are not doing it right. Maybe they feel they are just venting and not addressing any of their problems. Other patients are overwhelmed by the amount of homework, or they are distressed that their therapist seems strange to them. Sometimes they have been in therapy for many years, but are not sure it is helping. These worries are extremely common, and often a good sign. It is unfortunate for patients, but much of the therapeutic encounter is "behind the scenes". I am sure there are some bad therapists out there, content to charge for being a friend. However, having spoken about hundreds of cases with dozens of therapists, I would consider this rare and typically a misunderstanding of the process. Patients tell me they just talk about what is on their mind, and the therapist will tell me about recurrent themes, behavioral patterns in the room, reactivity to confrontation, burgeoning transference, and increased psychological mindedness about their condition.

Consequently, I find it hard to advise patients about who to see and what to do in therapy until I have spoken with the therapist about the case. Generally, I do think patients can be aware of common factors, empathy, shared goals, etc. If these are present, I suggest patients give the therapy some time to work. If they really feel strongly it is not helping, a discussion with the therapist can be an amazing tool. Sometimes the therapist will open up about the process, and other times the therapist will change methods. If all else fails, a conversation about frustrations in the therapy session can lead to a referral to someone who might match the patient's needs better.

When it comes to deciding on a therapist, it is a

good idea to start with understanding your goals. Do you want to work on a particular symptom like panic attacks? Do you want to clean up your habits, since all of your doctors seem to know what you are doing wrong, but not how to do it better? Maybe you want to be at peace with a new reality of life, knowing that your old way of living is no longer possible. Maybe your symptoms are mild, and you are beginning to feel a looming distaste with the life you have built, like you are living for others rather than yourself. Using the overviews of different approaches in this chapter, you might be able to scan through advertisements for therapists and either identify key words or how their language feels, and use this to pick who might be a good match.

It's not that simple, though, is it? The ads online never seem to say they take your insurance. Most of them are listed as not taking new clients, or they put you on a waitlist when you call and give no indication when they might give you an appointment. Maybe you can apply to a corporate group, but they will just assign some random therapist to you. Finding a therapist is an impossible task, made all the more impossible by how tired you are. It can be so frustrating, and with so many barriers, it can be easy to give up. No one would blame you. We all know how hard it is. Just say that you are on a few wait lists, and most doctors will praise you for the effort and resume care without it. But please consider trying again, getting on another wait list, or finding someone out of network even though it will take extra forms to get reimbursed.

I cannot impress upon you how vital it can be to the treatment team, and how most of the failures in care come from neglecting this component. I have had patients who went to ten different physical therapists because it "wasn't working" until they found one who injects a bit of psychological treatment into the physical therapy session. They are amazed, suddenly their bodies are behaving. Convincing the patient that those 2 minutes of untrained advice per PT session might be inferior to a dedicated professional psychologist is surprisingly difficult. At the end, all I can do is continue to softly encourage people to try again. You deserve help. With up front effort, checking on the waitlist status, sending out a few more inquiries, and sending an email and calling, success is a lot more likely. After you find someone you like, it gets much easier.

CHAPTER 8: WHAT ELSE CAN BE DONE?

While the majority of modern Western medicine focuses on surgeries, medications, and Western physical therapies, the unspoken truth is that the most important components to health are often neglected in the consulting room. There are a few reasons for this, but it has been disastrous in our medical system. We are living longer, but we are living sicker. We add more and more medications to cover the symptoms, but in many cases we are not addressing the causes of illness.

In this chapter, I hope to explain a broad scope of some different ways patients can improve their symptoms and overall health. It is, however, important to come to this from the right perspective. Just like there is no magic pill or even the right pill for all patients, there is no right combination of interventions for everyone. It is best to initially see this as a menu of options to consider rather than get overwhelmed by thinking they must all be done. Moreover, some things like sleep hygiene or searching for dietary triggers can be a life-long process of gradual adjustments.

The two major things that must be kept in mind are 1. there is no exact right way for someone to approach these changes, and 2. a person cannot and should not try to do everything. Trying to do everything will be exhausting and often depressing. If someone makes too many changes all at once, they cannot be sure which individual change had what impact. It is also very worrisome when a patient comes to me for a second visit and they say they "did everything" we discussed since I know that is impossible. Usually they did a couple things for each area, often only for a few days.

Sleep hygiene is often the first thing patients are sure they have mastered, but with thousands of potential interventions I know it is not likely they have done everything. I have only known one person who got close, and she was extremely neurotic about the topic. She and her husband bought a house specifically because it had a perfect room, in the center of the house, without windows, just large enough for her bed, and no electrical plugs. No electrical devices (or her husband) were allowed in that room, and she had a 3 hour nighttime ritual to help her fall asleep. While she did work, she had a very strict schedule for the whole day designed around her sleep hygiene. Do not do that, but also do not imagine there is a quick way to finish any of the topics in this chapter and "get them out of the way".

The last thing to remember before indulging in this chapter is that these are the hardest treatments available for two reasons: 1. They are almost entirely about changing daily routines. It takes 2 seconds to take a pill, 30 minutes to do an exercise, and an hour to do psychotherapy. Changing daily routines, on the other hand, can take almost continuous thoughtfulness and retraining that can affect most of your waking time. 2. These treatments require a lot of strategizing, and finding help with this is much harder than getting an appointment with a physical therapist. There are thousands of psychotherapists in a given state, but only a small handful will specialize in sleep therapy. There are many nutritionists in any given city, but many of them will have a very limited focus, not truly understanding the complex needs of Long Covid patients. With tens of millions affected by Long Covid, there just are not enough therapy providers to give patients individualized help determining a good routine. However, there are copious online resources, books, and guides to help patients do the work independently and more stable providers like therapists have many tools to keep patients motivated and organized.

Sleep Is Key

Likely the most high-yield intervention, able to give the most patients the most benefit, is working to improve sleep quality. While there are definitely plenty of people with pure insomnia syndromes, far more people sleep a reasonable number of hours but have poor sleep quality. This happens in the extreme with sleep apnea or severe PTSD, but the average person has erratic sleep cycles for the simple reason that their brain does not know when nighttime is. Our brains were designed to key off of our daily experiences to adjust to a 24-hour sleep-wake cycle. Our brains want sunlight first thing in the morning, but other than TV and fluorescent lighting, many of us have little exposure to the sun. Throughout any given day, we have a bright lightbulb sitting above our heads telling us it is constantly noon. Our brains want to see the sunset and have about 3-4 hours to prepare for bed, but we watch TV shows with flashing lights right until we want our brains to sleep. We read books or watch TV laying in bed, and when we decide to sleep, our brains ask "where's the book, where's the TV?" Consequently, if people are hooked up to EEG, the textbook pattern of slowly going into deep sleep and slowly going into shallow sleep throughout the night is rare.

My experience is that there are two main objections to starting sleep work. The first is simply, "I sleep fine" followed by a nice story of sleeping 8 hours and feeling generally well rested (even if they need a pot of coffee to make it to work). The other response, surprising to me for the first 20 or so times I heard it, is "It's ok, I'm a non-sleeper." These patients are convinced that their bodies only ever need 2-3 hours of sleep per night. Both of these perspectives are very hard to overcome because they are fixed beliefs these patients have and there is little time in a clinical encounter to try to convince them otherwise. However, I have definitely had "fine sleepers" and "non-sleepers" who finally consented to get treatment. With some initial effort, they were able to get significant improvement in their symptoms with some simple changes to their sleep habits. The truth is, they were living life for so long in a half-daze they did not really know what being awake felt like. When they finally got to experience wakefulness for the first time, they quickly became true believers This is seen most dramatically in some patients with obstructive sleep apnea. Some patients will report that within a week or two they feel like they are 20 years younger after starting a CPAP machine at night.

There are specialized psychologists who use a form of cognitive behavioral therapy designed for insomnia (CBT-I). They use a variety of interventions including charting behaviors and sleep, finding achievable goals, and helping to find strategies to reach them. However, there are not enough well-trained insomnia specialists to go around. I find starting with an online review of the Sleep Foundation website to be a reasonable starting point. A simple search on Google for "sleep hygiene" will direct you to articles, videos, and books on the topic. Of the myriad books on sleep, my patients have responded well to <u>Say Goodnight</u>

<u>to Insomnia</u> because it is so simply written with practical advice. However, there is no comprehensive resource that gives all of the available tools, so after patients tell me they have "done everything", I try to help them find more.

After ruling out other contributors to poor sleep quality like sleep apnea with your doctor, improving sleep always starts with an honest survey of habits and patterns. Below is an example of a step-by-step program to clean up your sleep and improve your nighttime health.

Step 1: Every night write down when you go to bed, when you wake up, and a rough estimation of how long you think you stared at the ceiling and how many times you woke up. This may sound easy, but getting into this habit can be very difficult.

Step 2: Decide on a specific "down-time" and "up-time" that you can make as consistent as possible. No "catching up on the weekends" because an erratic sleep cycle is a bad sleep cycle.

Step 3: Implement an insomnia protocol. Generally, laying and staring at the ceiling is counterproductive if it lasts more than about 20 minutes. Instead, go to a separate room with soft lighting and do something simple like read a silly book and sip on warm water or caffeine-free tea for 15 minutes. Then try to go to bed again.

Step 4: Create an evening ritual (not in the bedroom), done every night, that may last between 30 minutes and an hour, or even longer. This wind-down time should be very consistent and not include anything stimulating. Reading is much better than watching TV because your brain can slowly reduce the speed of your reading while TV or music usually drives the pace. Some people add a meditation or a prayer, where others do a stretching or breathing routine or drink a nighttime tea (ginger, lemon balm, chamomile, or valerian root are common). This should be tailored to your personality.

Step 5: Search for inappropriate habits throughout the day and slowly reduce them. Caffeine should have a hard endpoint in the day. Some people can have caffeine till around 2pm, but many people benefit from stopping at noon or before. No sugary drinks, especially after 2-3pm. Alcohol may seem to help people fall asleep, but it (and many sedatives) actually ruins the sleep quality. A good rule of thumb is to not feel any of the effects of alcohol at least an hour before bedtime. Mid-day exercise is important for sleep quality, but evening exercise is stimulating if done after around 5pm.

Step 6: Make all other habits as consistent as possible. If you drink coffee, drink alcohol, or smoke marijuana, doing a lot one day and very little the next will wreck your sleep quality. Exercising heavily for 5 days and then taking days off will confuse your cycle. Eating big meals every other day will confuse your whole metabolic system. Apart from work, each day should roughly resemble the next.

Step 7: Do a deep search for patterns. Some foods (especially nighttime foods) can make it far more difficult to fall asleep. Some people may wind you up and make it difficult to settle into a nighttime routine.

Step 8: Make the bedroom sacred. Ideally, the bedroom should be for sleep and sex only. Some people say sleep only, but that is ridiculous because sex is a very important part of nighttime mental and physical health. Getting rid of anything that could trigger you to start planning for the next day or distract you should be removed. No cell phones or laptops, no bright lights. Dark curtains and soothing images only.

Step 9: Take a slow deep breath and realize there is always more to do, but no one is perfect. If you have been able to achieve a fraction of the above, you have already done more than the majority of people out there. What you have done will be good for your mental health, your heart, and your brain, and you should be applauded even if you had failures along the way.

Step 10: Go back to step 1 and start the process

all over again, because you can always do more, and it will always help your symptoms and your health.

I know this may sound exhausting, or perhaps boring. Making every day exactly the same, no alcohol before bed, and waking up early on weekends would have driven me crazy when I was younger. The good thing is that there are many simple bits of advice that can be fun and relaxing with very little effort. Also, it can't be All or None. Every little bit helps with any individual intervention having some positive impact on sleep quality. This is not the case with medications, which must be titrated very specifically and must be taken every day to work at all. Often patients will start by having the same ginger tea and a melatonin at the same time every evening. Others may start with a light therapy box (search online for "10,000 lux" to find a few options) for 30 minutes each morning (obviously not when migraine is the biggest issue). They have even begun making very effective glasses for light therapy (I have enjoyed the Luminette brand light therapy glasses). These baby steps can work wonders and motivate patients to make further adjustments over time.

Diet And Nutrition

With all of the physicians I have known, counseling around diet and nutrition seems to be the most vital, the most neglected, and the most difficult task for them. It is also the hardest intervention to study in most of our chronic illnesses. The importance of nutrition has not always been so universally accepted, and some of the biggest nutrition researchers in Western medicine will give horror stories about being laughed off of the stage at their conventions. Dean Ornish is a good example. He would tell stories about presenting data to a room full of cardiologists and the room becoming nearly empty by the time he finished his presentation. At the time, the world was so excited about the slight delay in cardiovascular disease with statin medications they had little interest in hearing about diet changes. When Ornish presented his data on plaques in the heart vessels actually shrinking with a holistic diet-based approach, they thought he had fabricated his data.

Nowadays, many cardiologists will say that they fully believe strict dietary measures are at least as useful as drugs, but why bother when patients will not do it. At best, cardiologists will give a handout describing their preferred diet (DASH, Mediterranean, etc...) and let the patient decide if they will throw it away in the first trash can they see or if they will wait and throw it away when they get home. And cardiology is not alone. While clear scientific data is limited, anecdotal evidence abounds. I have spoken with oncologists who believe that a strict diet is more likely to delay or reverse cancer growth than their heavy chemotherapeutic drugs. I have known rheumatologists who believe diet would be more effective than their $80K per year biologic medicines. I have discussed nutrition with psychiatrists who believe that ADHD would not exist if pizza and hotdogs were outlawed. Universally, practitioners say diet is either ignored in their consult room, or they just remind patients they should "eat healthier foods".

I have also met a few physicians who would give their advice firmly, clearly, and directly. This is not necessarily better. When discussing diet with my own primary care doctor due to elevated cholesterol, I was asked if I had heard of the 2, 2, and 2 rule (I had not). Her advice regarding meat intake was to only eat two small servings of fish per week, two small servings of chicken per month, and two small servings of red meat or pork per year. This did not change my behavior because it was so far removed from my normal routine as to seem absurd. It would probably have been easier for me to receive a recommendation for abandoning meat entirely rather than to follow the 2, 2, and 2 rule.

Other physicians seem to jump onto every new fad. For some time, doctors were regularly recommending intermittent fasting or the Atkins diet because they were in the news a lot and had some animal data that might have been encouraging. However, the subtleties of nutritional counseling are very complex. It does not help that most physicians have never had any formal training in either nutrition or behavioral counseling. This is why I have met a lot of confused migraineurs who told me they got much worse after a doctor recommended intermittent fasting (which is terrible for migraine) and even a few stroke patients on an Atkins diet that had LDL (bad cholesterol) higher than the lab test could read.

The reality is, most fad diets are healthy for some people and terrible for others. Unfortunately, there is no one-size-fits-all with nutritional counseling, and much of that has to do with the personality of the patient. Ideally, this discussion would include dietary counseling with the purpose of finding achievable goals, tempering expectations, and slowly shifting to more healthy diets over time. Some people are very motivated by quick results, but this needs to be matched with some plan to ensure long-term sustainability. Others will be able to tolerate baby steps in the right direction even though the results will come with a delay. For many, food is so enmeshed in cultural identification there really needs to be a family meeting or community meeting to find ways for the whole community to eat in a more healthy and sustainable way.

Before I give too many specific recommendations, I also want to emphasize the important role food can have for some people. There is an enormous amount of shame and trauma related to food and body image. This is extraordinarily common, and typically neglected even in mental health consultations. In my opinion, patients should never feel shame about food or their body. The shame is on our society and the profession of medicine that these patients are not given access to appropriate treatment and are further traumatized by stigma related to weight and appearance. I have had many chronic pain and chronic fatigue patients who had nearly abandoned engaging with medical treatments due to physicians overtly fat shaming them. Maybe they spent 10 years struggling with anorexia and in the end their body settled a bit above the recommended BMI. Perhaps they had a severe depression syndrome and the only medications that helped caused severe weight gain. When a doctor tells them "you'd be fine if you just lost some weight," it is a crushing blow to their spirit. All of the below recommendations can be misinterpreted as guidance on weight loss, and could trigger patients who have been traumatized by physicians who were not as aware of the suffering caused by anorexia, bulimia, and orthorexia. I do not intend that, and it is very reasonable to skip the rest of this section if it might cause discomfort.

Below is a generalized guideline, and it may not be appropriate for every person. Ideally, meeting with a nutritionist is a good idea, but keep in mind that they may or may not be good at taking a patient-centered approach in a non-biased way. Typically their advice will be good, but they may insist on an all-in approach for a patient that needs baby steps or vice versa. However, the reason to have a nutritionist is to consider any red flags in a patient's approach and to keep patients motivated.

Step 1: Think globally about your current and past

dietary patterns. What has worked in the past in changing diet, for how long, and which dietary changes have not worked.

Step 2: Truly and honestly decide if you are an "all-in" or a "baby step" personality. This should be what has worked in the past, not what you wish you could be.

Step 3: Write down foods you love, hate, and can or cannot live without.

Step 4: Search online for DASH Diet, Mediterranean diet, green mediterranean diet, anti-inflammatory diet, macrobiotic diet, and consider reading a book on the Ornish approach. This is to help you learn about some of the different "healthy diet" guides out there.

Step 5: Search online for "Migraine elimination diets" and "Migraine food triggers" to learn about "trigger foods" that are more likely to exacerbate certain symptoms (but for each person only a few will).

Step 6: Spend a few weeks truly analyzing what you put in your mouth- meals, snacks, drinks, everything. This can be on a calendar, a book, or otherwise.

Step 7: Consider barriers like who eats or cooks in the same household, if you have the ability to bring food to work, or if you really hate to cook.

Step 8: Consider how to overcome barriers, like can everyone in the house eat healthier, make cooking a fun family process, etc...

Step 9: Make a decision that you think will be an achievable goal, and come up with a plan to organize your time around food to make it possible.

Step 10: Reassess - what is working, what is failing, and what could make it easier to succeed.

I also consider there to be a few fundamental "Rules" when designing a healthy diet. These, again, are not universal, but they have worked for most of my patients most of the time.

Rule 1: Any diet should be sustainable. If you think you can only do it for a short period, it is not the right diet for you.

Rule 2: If any particular food item makes you feel sluggish and ill within 6 hours after eating it, it should not be on the list. Even healthy foods can be triggers.

Rule 3: It is harder to eat what is not in the house than things in the house, so the shopper must be on board.

Rule 4: The first 3 days of any diet are the hardest, the first three weeks are the strangest, and after 3 months, it becomes a habit.

Rule 5: "Healthy diets" can be made unhealthy. Trying to make vegan pizza your only source of calories is unhealthy.

Rule 6: Variety is essential for nutrition. If you find that you eat the exact same category of vegetable and never try new things, you are likely missing vital nutrients.

Rule 7: Supplements are typically safe and sometimes necessary, like B12 for vegetarians, but some can be toxic. Talk to a nutritionist or a doctor about any supplements.

Rule 8: Your energy is an economy. Calories in with food, out with exercise. If neither calorie intake nor exercise change, weight usually will not.

Rule 9: Rapid weight loss is almost universally bad for the body. I would rather someone consistently lose 1 pound per month than 12 pounds every other month.

Rule 10: If a food is heavily processed, or if it is prepared by someone else, it is most likely unhealthy even if it seems to be mostly vegetables. You can put just as much butter on veggies as you can on meat.

Generally, following these steps and rules are more important than which diet you choose. A final rule is that food should be pleasurable. Given, if someone avoids sugar for a few weeks healthier foods will become more tasty, but if you think that you are resigned to either "be healthy and sad" or "be unhealthy and happy", your diet will fail.

I will not pretend to know how each diet truly affects Long COVID specifically other than to say there is great data on various diets and their effects on nearly every body system, and every Long COVID symptom. Inflammation markers clearly change based on diet. The bacteria in the gut, which change with dietary changes, have been linked to many severe diseases and neurologic disorders as well as immune system disorders. While there are many interesting theories related to how these connections work, there are no convincing theories that would modify the simple recommendations we give in medicine. The key is just to do it, adjust when needed, and stay motivated. Finding how to stay motivated is the hardest part for most patients, and when you find your motivation, hold onto it.

Building Social Infrastructure

Most of the effects of Long COVID can be isolating, leading to a cycle of reduced engagement with friendships. This often starts with people who glean most of their social activity from work. Old, enjoyable friendships can drift away if the symptoms limit one's ability to engage with those people. Finances play a key role at times, with expensive hobbies becoming impractical while on disability. It can be hard to justify spending time with friends when you feel you do not have enough energy to bathe half of the time. Maybe you feel like you canceled with a good friend a few times and now you feel ashamed to reach out again. Perhaps you feel they just pity you, and you want to be seen as the strong person you once were. However it happens, most people with post-viral fatigue syndromes find their life shrinking and shrinking until it is just them, their bed, and their Grubhub account.

Most of the literature discussing the therapeutic benefit of friendships and hobbies is in the field of psychology. Isolating in depression is thought by many evolutionary psychologists to be a natural process to protect the tribe. If the sick/depressed person stays active they are a drain on the community resources, but if they stay isolated then the community can continue without them. However, we no longer live in tribes where someone who cannot hunt or farm is a drain on the tribe to be abandoned or institutionalized.

We know that many of these people can be treated and can return to a productive life. Some of the most beloved artists and creative minds throughout history had spells of deep depression. People get better, and people have intrinsic value beyond their ability to hunt and gather. The interesting thing is how the cycle can be interrupted by "behavioral activation" and socialization, even without curing the underlying depression or illness. I should emphasize that people have so many unique traits that affect this. The two most important are related to habits and beliefs developed in childhood, and whether a person is an introvert or an extrovert.

In childhood, someone may have been told (or more often shown) that someone is successful if they devote themselves to work. Others had an emphasis placed on success in sports, intellectual pursuits, or the ability to take care of others. While having goals and values like these can be great in normal circumstances, when that most valuable skill is taken away by Long COVID, it is extraordinarily hard to feel like life is meaningful. It is also particularly difficult to retrain a value system. We are wired to think (or at the very least society tells us) we have value when what we do has value. I would not want people to think what we do does not matter, but if only one activity has value and that is taken away, we must reframe our thoughts to survive.

Eventually, nearly everyone can find something they are capable of that they believe has value, but this is an exhausting search. Trying out new hobbies or training new skills is hard enough without severe brain fog and fatigue. In the meantime, I find it is important for people to begin to believe they have inherent value that is not defined by what they can do right now. For some, a focus on prior successes can give them a sense of personal value and they have "earned" the right to rest and take care of themselves.

For others, they must accept they have intrinsic value as a person, and all people deserve to live and enjoy their life. For some this may sound simple and obvious, but childhood is full of false dichotomies, motivational statements, and unforced conflicts that live in the subconscious and are difficult to re-write.

Regarding introversion/extroversion, there are many theoretical approaches. For the purposes of healing after Long COVID and building a social infrastructure, there are two main models I find appropriate. One is related to which situations recharge you, and the other has to do with where you like to spend your energy. If both functions are extroverted (E/E), then the biggest trouble is navigating ways to have fun with people since you enjoy it and are recharged by the energy of others. If both functions are introverted (I/I), the difficulty is finding ways to stay mentally and physically active without being around too many groups, often with a few close individual friendships being key. As an I/E, I need plenty of personal time to recharge, but must get some social activity to enjoy my life. People who are E/I, while rare, need to have one or two major social events per week and then lots of personal time for hobbies and tasks to have fun and feel productive. Figuring out this personality component is vital in designing a new social infrastructure.

The second goal is to take an honest assessment of your current activities, your activities prior to COVID, and activities from younger life. What tasks give or gave you joy, and which seemed more draining than supportive? Did you have any hobbies or friendships that you pushed aside for work? Was there a skill you enjoyed when you were younger that you could repurpose into a new daily activity you can tolerate despite your fatigue? Did you have a goal or aspiration as a child such as music or art that was never pursued because your parents told you to focus on school instead? These can be great resources to determine which new hobbies might fill your time.

Generically, you want to think of your energy and identity as supported by various pillars. If one is pulled out, you need to have enough to stay upright. A three or four legged stool will fall over if one leg breaks. A 12 legged stool may seem ridiculous, but you could remove four or five legs and it will probably never collapse. Each hobby, each relationship, and each interest is a value, where any one of them falling away should not impact your self-esteem or your joy in life.

After completing an honest assessment of current and previous hobbies, I recommend people come up with a game plan they think will be achievable. Doing too much all at once is often counterproductive, but adding in one or two new pillars every other week is a more sustainable approach. The first week, maybe schedule a couple phone calls or lunch dates with some old friends. See which friends are easy to talk to, and try not to focus on only negative topics. Be honest about not doing well, but try to turn the conversation to happier times or hopes for the future. This takes practice, but most people do not want to develop an identity as the "broken friend". Come up with a list of possible hobbies and get the materials to start doing them by week 3. Do not pressure yourself to do anything too hard at first, and do not give up if you fail. Rather than spend a thousand dollars on painting supplies, start with a simple palate of paints and a couple of canvasses. Rather than buying a grand piano, start with a cheap keyboard. It can be very frustrating if you invest too much of your money or yourself in something that does not end up being a positive experience.

Consider building a social infrastructure to be like exercise. You have to practice, and it gets easier with time. You have to re-train your habits, which are often set in early adolescence. You have to gradually increase stamina. During the first few weeks or months, you will probably find barriers, make mistakes, or exhaust yourself by doing too much of a task that does not really fit your personality type or by doing too much of one that would be more helpful in smaller doses. This sort of troubleshooting is a skill that also must be developed, just like painting or socializing.

Lastly, when deciding on which hobbies or friends to engage with, make sure they involve as much of your body, mind, and senses as possible. Cooking with people is a good example because it involves touch, smell, taste, physical exertion, and talking. While being alone and setting up a crockpot meal is much easier, it does not engage the other senses or mental activities. Reading a book is a wonderful hobby, but reading a book with a friend or writing reviews for fun is often more enriching. In this way, you can gradually combine hobbies and friendships to use more of your brain and body over time as you build stamina and skill.

Gadgets And Other Interventions

Patients are increasingly asking me about some of the other tools and techniques being marketed for some of the symptoms present in Long COVID. While none of them have been properly tested in Long COVID specifically, the data on their use in patients with similar symptom clusters is increasing. Below I will review some of the most common ones and discuss possible benefits and limitations of their use in patients with Long COVID.

Transcutaneous Electrical Nerve Stimulation (TENS) has been used in pain management for many decades. There are now a dozen different types, with deeper more complex electrical signals like an "Interferential TENS unit" showing greater efficacy, but at greater financial cost. The theories on how TENS treatments work have changed over the years. Initially, the idea was to locally soothe the tissue by giving it a distraction signal at the site of the injury. Since then, there have been studies on how electrical stimulation reduces inflammatory signals being sent down the nerves, interrupts the pain by activating the spinal cord or even higher in the brain (called sensory gating), and even encouraging healthy nerve growth. There is evidence for and against each of these theories, but because TENS units are so subjectively helpful and inexpensive, I think all patients should consider using them for limb or back pain with the guidance of a physician or physical therapist.

Steroid and other injections for joint and soft tissue pain have been used for almost a hundred years. I have found the pattern of data has always followed a similar trajectory. The initial data is always very encouraging, with patients reporting reduced pain and increased functionality. Later data shows that some people get better, many people experience benefits that do not last more than a few days, and some people report feeling worse. Later, especially with steroids, a study will show long-term harm when done repeatedly. The reality is that if the right patients are chosen, for the right condition, injection of steroid, analgesic, or other chemicals should help quickly and last for weeks to months at minimum. Unfortunately, patients must rely on the wisdom and experience of their physicians to determine if steroid injections would help them and this can be deeply frustrating.

Cold laser therapy has been of interest to medical researchers for many decades, but it was not until the early 2000s that the first studies showed it was safe and effective in some patients. Theories abound for how it works, including a change in local inflammatory processes, changes to blood vessel growth, and stimulation of other soft tissue cells. Having read the literature thoroughly, I can say that much of it is speculation. It has yet to become standard practice in the majority of the Western medical world, and there is a lot of very well-intentioned skepticism about its use. It is rarely covered by insurance, and is mostly used by alternative medicine providers or chiropractors, but has also been adopted by many people who should not be practicing medicine at all. Patients can usually tell if they are seeing a good alternative medicine provider or a snake oil salesman by how it is presented. If someone tells you it is definitely going to help because it is "calibrated to the frequency of the COVID-19 virus", then they are making things up and any further advice from that provider should be avoided.

Electrical stimulation to the head comes in many different intensities and flavors, and has been a hot topic in mood disorders, migraine, and even epilepsy. The oldest validated treatment is, of course, electroconvulsive therapy. While ECT got a lot of negative press from fictional accounts like the movie *One Flew Over the Cuckoo's Nest* and groups like Scientologists, the reality is it is a very safe and often life-saving intervention. Severe depression that has not responded to medication and talk therapy will be significantly improved (often completely resolved) with ECT in about 90% of patients. Most of the criticisms related to cognitive side effects came from an individual very biased researcher, and most people return to normal cognitive functioning within a month of finishing treatment. It was more dangerous, potentially, before we learned how to properly sedate people, but now it is known to be safer for long-term functioning than most of the medications we prescribe for depression.

Lesser forms of electrical stimulation such as those used for depression, brain fog, and anxiety are called TDCS (Transcutaneous Direct Current Stimulation), which is still in the process of being validated and improved. I expect it will become a standard treatment option in the future because it is cheap and can have very positive impacts on certain symptoms. Its pop-culture fame comes from a small study in 2013 where soldiers were found to have better focus, stamina, and visuospatial accuracy after a short course of TDCS. There was a popular *Radiolab* podcast episode about it in 2014, which is enjoyable and does include the frightening potential consequences if done without medical guidance. Many "brain hackers" were building their own TDCS devices. Some were developing mania and one went temporarily blind. This therapy should be directly guided by a physician who has experience with neuromodulation.

Other devices with even lower levels of electrical stimulation are readily available on the market. There are four different wearable devices that are FDA approved for the treatment of migraine. Very small amounts of electrical stimulation to the trigeminal nerve (usually on the forehead) can have a modest but meaningful impact on migraine headache symptoms. Other devices used on the ear or neck can stimulate the Vagus nerve, which is very important in the brain/body feedback loop in anxiety. These devices are validated and FDA approved for panic with or without PTSD.

Lastly, magnets in medicine have been used (often inappropriately) since the 1700s. The most famous scoundrel to cure people by waving magnets around was Franz Mesmer (where we get the term mesmerize) and his dancing around in a robe with magnets did not help patients. Any benefit would have been placebo, or hypnosis if I am being generous. However, modern medicine has revived magnet therapy over the past 30 years with a treatment called Transcranial Magnetic Stimulation (TMS). This uses a very strong magnet that can create a small electrical current in underlying brain tissue to help disrupt or amplify certain brain networks. Better devices with more complex settings are coming out every year, and the treatment is currently approved for treatment-resistant depression. The current research is showing it may also have unique benefits for many neurologic conditions including Tourette's, Parkinson's, and others. It may also help improve recovery from stroke and traumatic brain injury. Unfortunately, while the results are "statistically significant" the effect size is not always. Where ECT resolves depression in most cases, TMS reduces the symptoms modestly. With a treatment protocol that is 5 days per week for at least a month, it is also extremely inconvenient for many, and the cost of the machines make the total cost between $50,000-$70,000 for an individual treatment course. I rarely recommend TMS since less time-consuming and less costly treatments with better data for efficacy (like Ketamine infusions and ECT) exist.

What Should I Do?

The answer to this question is different from person to person. In the next chapter I will discuss an ideal coordinated medical approach for Long COVID care. It is important to know the breadth of potential interventions out there, as to avoid the hopelessness that comes from a lack of options. However, spending millions of dollars jumping down every rabbit hole is often harmful. A simple but broad approach is much better for the majority of patients. It is so disturbing when I meet patients who have seen a thousand specialists that have spent a year evaluating every possible cancer, inflammatory disease, nutritional deficiency, and hormone imbalance instead of treating the obvious problems the patient brought to their PCP.

I tend to recommend patients focus on the basics first. Are there any medical conditions such as hypertension, hypothyroidism, or life-long depression that have not been fully treated? Are there safe and effective treatments for the Long COVID symptoms that have not been tried, like those used for migraine, fatigue, or depression? Is there any way to optimize overall health through sleep, diet, exercise, and socialization? Only after these basics are covered should patients and their primary providers be worried about experimental lasers or start looking for super rare medical conditions. New things can be fun, but relying on experimental treatments or expensive gadgets is a fool's errand, no matter how much the internet promises that the next new miracle is on the horizon. My patients and I cannot wait for the horizon to get here, and my hope is that by following a few simple protocols, they will not have to.

CHAPTER 9: THE JOURNEY FOR HELP

When patients enter my office, they are often broken and afraid. They might have seen three or four doctors who told them nothing was wrong, or perhaps just their PCP who thought something neurological might be happening. Their response to me asking how I can help them is frequently, "fix me" or an immediate and lengthy diatribe about the thousand symptoms they have had over the past few months. Beginning to wade into their history is a humbling experience, learning deep and intimate details about someone's suffering when they were a complete stranger only moments ago. Studies show that doctors will typically interrupt this spontaneous narrative within about 2 minutes to probe or correct patients, but I often let patients continue until they feel they are done. This approach has allowed them to get through the basic data (typically more than I need to make a diagnosis) and transition to more dynamic frustrations about the medical care they have been given so far. Even though I completely empathize with this, I have little to no control over the problems they are describing. They will often spend more time expressing frustrations over navigating the medical system than frustration over the symptoms of their disease. I am not a social worker or a case manager. I do not know much about their insurance company and why they refuse to cover standard treatments. At times, I get enough information from the referral documents to know how their PCP billed for the appointment, but nothing about the primary care doctor's other plans or thoughts.

In this chapter, I will overview an ideal approach. I do not want patients to feel frustrated by how disorganized their care has been, but I hope that a review of the different potential options will help them look back and fill in the gaps. It is important to understand that this is just an example of an approach and not a guideline for all patients or all physicians. What physicians do is often standard of care based on their best medical knowledge, and not any sort of malpractice or neglect. It is unfortunate, but with most chronic illnesses, including Long COVID, patients must take a major role in advocating for themselves. With little medical training, this is unreasonable to ask of patients, but that does not make it untrue. It is my hope that this book, and this chapter specifically, will help patients to set up the right team, check off the right boxes, and get the treatment that will help them feel better.

Is This Long COVID?

I have discussed Long COVID at length, but I
have not really addressed how to determine if
you have this particular syndrome. Many patients
developed symptoms similar to Long COVID before
the pandemic, and there are many reasons for this.
While COVID has some unique effects on the lungs
and heart, the combination of chronic fatigue, pain,
depression, dizziness, migraine, and other symptoms
can occur for many reasons. We have discussed a
similar syndrome that occurs after mono-nucleosis
(Epstein-Barr virus) and Lyme disease. Some people
seem to develop it spontaneously without a known
infection, but many theorists believe a mild infection
occurs that is not really noticed. This is seen in other
post-infectious, immune-mediated neurological
disorders like Guillain-Barre syndrome and acute
demyelinating encephalomyelitis. In the typical time
course for a post-infectious inflammatory disorder,
symptoms occur around 3 weeks after the infection,
but there is a wide range. Some patients have
symptoms within a week and some have symptoms
starting a couple of months after the infection.

Long COVID is a bit different, but it is because
researchers decided to make it that way. Some
committee somewhere has decided that Long COVID

does not exist until symptoms have been present for three months, so all the research will be based on a three month follow-up after diagnosis. However, it is not entirely unreasonable since many patients have complete resolution of symptoms without treatment before the three month follow-up. Symptoms within the first three weeks are considered to be due to the active infection and the inflammation the body uses to fight the infection. Any symptoms that start after the initial infection but within three months would be considered a different diagnosis entirely. Currently, those symptoms are the "Post-Acute Sequelae of COVID" (or PASC). This is an arbitrary distinction, but it is how the research is categorizing symptoms and that has some very important consequences. All medications used to treat Long COVID will not be tested for safety and efficacy before three months post-infection.

My patients typically describe the classic post-infectious timeline. The infection lasts days to a week, and within a week or two after that the new symptoms started. Often fatigue or migraine symptoms dominate. These slowly escalate over the next month and then stabilize. These patients have a hard time describing the exact timeline and which symptoms occur when, but by the three month mark they typically have their complete syndrome with a cycle of insomnia, worsening migraine, worsening fatigue, and worsening depression. They already feel hopeless by three months, which is reasonable after over two months of misery. The unfortunate message is that until the three month mark, the symptoms are considered PASC, and for the unforeseeable future, all of the research and guidelines will say there is nothing to do but wait.

The good news is that many patients have complete (or near complete) resolution of all symptoms by that point. By all means, see a doctor in the meantime for advice and to discuss symptoms. Definitely call 911 or go to the emergency department if you think you might be having any sort of medical emergency like a stroke or a heart attack. However, if symptoms are stable, the goal needs to be to see your PCP as soon as you can after the 3 month mark to start the process of getting diagnosed and finding appropriate treatments. In the meantime, work on sleep, diet, exercise, and any other global health measures you can think of.

Primary Care Is Primary For A Reason

The first step after determining you might have Long COVID is to create a close relationship with your Primary Care Physician. Even if they know very little about the disorder, PCP offices are designed to be the hub from which all other medical care should be directed. Our society tells us that super-specialists are "better" in some way, but no super-specialist has the knowledge or infrastructure to determine in which order and in what way a doctor should take care of these patients. There are too many organ systems and physiologic processes affected by the COVID virus or the Long COVID syndrome. Unfortunately, many of my patients describe extreme frustration with their current PCP and tell me, "it is impossible to find a new PCP these days". This is not a problem with an easy solution, but every other problem in seeking help for Long COVID will be twice as hard to fix without a PCP to help herd the cats.

At the PCP appointment, it is important to have both an open mind and direct goals. You should gather everything you know about your past medical history (including any odd previous symptoms that were never diagnosed), family history, prior medications with doses and how they affected you, as well as a timeline of how symptoms have changed since you got sick. You do not need to flood the doctor with all of this information, but having it readily available is key so your doctor can help you decide what to do. Whole books could be written on how patients could better navigate their medical appointments, but a few principles can moderate expectations and help make them more productive.

1. Write down everything you hope to achieve, and any questions you have, and bring it with you. Any good doctor will give at least 5 minutes at the end of an encounter for an "Anything else?" type question.

2. Expect some initial lab work, especially if you

have not been there in a while. PCPs have important algorithms to make sure your kidneys, liver, hormones, and cardiovascular health are not an urgent concern.

3. Do not expect answers on day 1, but always insist on knowing the next steps if tests "come back normal". You want them to decide this during the appointment, not three weeks later when the last lab comes back within normal limits.

4. Make sure to have more frequent check-ups while you are still getting "worked up" so your PCP is aware of what the other doctors are doing, but make those check-ups after the specialist appointments so they can adjust course as needed.

5. Figure out if your PCP prefers electronic communication or phone calls, and expect that nurses will gather much of the info.

6. Sometimes Nurse Practitioners or Physician's Assistants can be far more effective at coordinating care and communicating with patients than the D.O. or M.D.

7. Don't assume the PCP team has access to everything your specialists tell you, or the tests they have ordered. Bring the labs, the imaging, and the prescription bottles with you.

Regardless of what your PCP says is going on, before you get to a specialist there are a few things you should organize. Having a folder to keep all of the questions, information, and answers together can be very helpful, especially with the disorganized brain fog of Long COVID. Having a family member or friend with you at all appointments can both help you organize your thoughts and advocate for your needs to be met. You should come to appointments with very specific goals, but be comfortable if the plan is different as long as your goals are voiced, heard, and will be addressed eventually, even if the PCP's plan does not resolve the problem. You should never insist the PCP order a test they do not want to order, but you should not forget that the test is a concern, and express why it is a concern to you. Finally, if the PCP does not give you a treatment for your symptoms (albeit after the initial tests), you should begin to voice a concern for a timeline or a referral. For example, if your symptoms are not better in 2 months, you want to know what to do or who to go to next.

This can be a very difficult negotiation for some PCPs, but it is often more dangerous if they seem happy to order a million tests and referrals all at once. The PCP may develop a condition called Ulysses syndrome where you run too many initial tests, a few tests come back positive, though unrelated to your original complaint, and they keep jumping down rabbit holes that lead nowhere. Ulysses (from Homer's *The Odyssey*) went on a simple journey, but each distraction led to another and he never made it home to his wife. If your doctor seems to have developed Ulysses syndrome, you may need to remind them why you reached out in the first place and to make sure they are still thinking about the symptoms you are most worried about.

In most cases, at the first visit a referral for some sort of physical treatment/therapy, psychotherapy, or both are helpful. If your cognition, mood, or insomnia symptoms are bothersome then establishing with a psychotherapist early is extremely important. If pain, fatigue, or stiffness is predominant in your syndrome, a physical therapist is key to start treatment and monitor progress. To be honest, even if pain and weakness are not the main symptoms, you may need a physical therapist to get you strong enough to tolerate traveling to so many appointments, and a psychotherapist to help you tolerate talking to so many physicians.

In short, it is your job to bring all of your information, keep your primary doctor focused on your concerns, and make sure any referrals actually happen and that the results from those referrals get back to your PCP. There will be some tests run by specialists that are best acted on by the PCP, like a neurologist ordering B12 and Thyroid studies when the PCP should guide treatment if abnormal. I recommend asking when the first set of test results will be available, or finding out when the specialist appointment is, and scheduling a PCP follow up within a month after that to keep progress moving.

Ruling Out/Treating Other Medical Contributors

Each PCP will have strengths and weaknesses. They may be great at managing blood pressure, but not at managing depression. They may have specialty training in pulmonology, but not know much about more complex disorders of metabolism. Luckily, most PCPs know this and will more quickly refer when a question is outside of their skill set. In this section, I will discuss common diseases that may contribute to the Long COVID syndrome, and which specialty manages them. Remember that most Long COVID patients do not have a severe lung disorder, endocrine disorder, or heart disorder, but seeing a specialist for these issues to discuss symptoms and rule out a few contributors is potentially quite helpful. Most people need few if any referrals, but when a referral is made, patients should know what the process could entail, which conditions the specialist should consider, and when to return to the PCP for next steps. Remember, when they say "the tests came back normal" it does not mean there is nothing wrong, even within the specialist's organ system. It typically does mean there is not anything serious and treatable in their organ system, so long as they have understood the patient's question. At that point, the PCP should have sufficient information regarding that medical discipline, or they may decide to get a second opinion if they are suspicious of a particular condition that was not evaluated.

Pulmonology

While much of the COVID syndrome and the Long COVID symptoms involve patients feeling short of breath, lung doctors only have a few major responsibilities when it comes to monitoring and treating either syndrome. In the early stages, they can look for any residual pneumonia or a handful of chronic respiratory problems like asthma or problems with the blood vessels in the lungs. They can also see if there are any residual changes on imaging of the lungs. While not always necessary, this often begins with an X-Ray of the lungs or a CT scan (which is simply a much clearer X-Ray where iodine contrast can be used to look at the blood vessels). Lung doctors may also order a Pulmonary Function Test (PFT) where a patient breathes deeply into a device to show how much air they can breathe in and out with a deep breath. This is as much a measure of the muscles around the lungs as the actual airways themselves. Between these few tests, and measures of oxygen or carbon dioxide during various activities, lung doctors can diagnose most of the disorders they are responsible for monitoring and treating.

Another thing a lung doctor should consider is a "sleep study". The key to getting a sleep study is to identify if you wake at night gasping, snore a lot, have a large neck, and/or are drowsy most of the day. The main set of questions they may ask related to daytime drowsiness are called the "Epworth Sleepiness Scale". I recommend looking up this scale before the appointment. Insurance companies will not pay for a sleep study unless you have an ESS score of 10 or more. As a neurologist, I order a lot of sleep studies and manage various forms of sleep apnea, but if the sleep apnea patient also has COPD, chronic lung inflammation, or some other severe lung disease, it is more appropriate for a lung doctor to be in charge so they can modify treatments and the CPAP oxygen requirements. At the end of the day, a sleep study is about deciding if a CPAP machine would be helpful and to diagnose a few neurologic conditions like narcolepsy, periodic limb movement disorder, or REM sleep behavior disorder. Unlike many other physicians, I ask patients up front if they think they would be able to tolerate a CPAP machine before I order the sleep study, and most people are willing to give it a try. After starting it, they feel so much better they typically persist until they are more comfortable with it.

Though pulmonologists are only responsible for ruling out a few major disorders, often present before contracting COVID, sleep apnea, asthma, COPD, and inflammatory lung disease are treatable disorders that can have a huge impact on Long COVID symptoms. If a lung doctor says the tests all came back normal, this is good and you can move on, but make sure they have considered these syndromes before leaving your last scheduled appointment with them.

Cardiology

While there are definitely some chronic lung diseases that affect Long COVID symptoms, shortness of breath after COVID is more often cardiac than pulmonary. The most common contributors to this are difficult to test for and not considered particularly dangerous, but on rare occasions when there is a serious heart rhythm problem or severe heart inflammation, it must be identified and treated quickly. Luckily, an EKG, a short term wearable heart monitor, and/or an ultrasound of the heart (Echocardiogram) can usually pick these up quickly.

Before meeting with a cardiologist, it is good to consider any chest symptoms like tightness, pain, heart racing, or feeling short of breath. It is also important to consider dizziness or feelings of lightheadedness that can occur if the heart or blood vessels are not pumping sufficient blood to the brain. Often more important, identify any patterns such as which symptoms occur together or in which order as well as what you do that brings on the symptom. With this information, the heart doctor can usually devise a plan to test for anything serious or treatable regarding the heart.

The POTS syndrome, typically treated by either neurology or cardiology, is particularly common in Long COVID, but few physicians in either field are truly comfortable diagnosing or treating it. The main diagnostic test is a tilt-table test. During this test, they use a table on a fulcrum to change a patient's position while they monitor the heart rate and observe any symptoms of lightheadedness or dizziness. Unfortunately, this can be positive in non-symptomatic individuals and can sometimes be normal in patients with classic POTS syndrome. This leaves interpretation and diagnosis in the hands of the physician, who may not even believe POTS is a real syndrome. After it is diagnosed, the treatment is difficult as well, though many medications can help a lot. Beta-blockers, SNRIs, mild steroids, salt tablets, and many others play a role. Additionally, drinking more water, wearing compression stockings or abdominal binders, and certain exercise and dietary regimens can reduce symptoms. However, I do want to emphasize that not all cardiologists are good at treating POTS, but all cardiologists should be good at quickly ruling out more life-threatening heart arrhythmias, heart failure, and heart inflammation that can cause similar symptoms. If you find yourself frustrated that the cardiologist says "everything is normal," and dismisses possible POTS, it is best not to rely on them to treat the condition.

Lastly, if symptoms are severe (loss of consciousness after chest symptoms), occur infrequently (less than once per week), and the initial testing is normal, it is important to consider an implantable loop monitor. Fundamentally, if you are not hooked up to a monitor during the symptoms, you cannot rule out a heart rhythm abnormality being the cause. I have had patients who had multiple cardiologists say nothing was wrong with their heart, but with an implantable loop monitor they found a severe heart rhythm problem that only occurred twice per year. A loop monitor is a small microchip placed under the skin of the chest that measures the heart's electrical activity, and it can be left in for years. The cardiologist places them (takes about 5 minutes) and a report is generated once per month via a wireless connection. You should have a device that allows you to "mark" periods with symptoms so the cardiologist can look very closely at that event.

In short, heart doctors should be responsible for ruling out life-threatening conditions like a heart attack, severe heart inflammation, or dangerous heart rhythm abnormalities. They will typically start with an EKG to look at the electrical activity of the heart at that moment, but can order a wearable 30-day monitor or place an implantable loop monitor to measure the heart's electrical activity during any fainting or spells of chest tightness or heart racing. They usually do not need to do much more in Long COVID, but some are good at treating symptoms of POTS. When they say "nothing is wrong" just realize they are saying that your heart is not wholly responsible for your symptoms, and there does not seem to be any cardiac reason to rush to the ER.

Endocrinology

My patients have had very mixed experiences with endocrinologists in the setting of the fatigue in Long COVID. One endocrinologist will run about 2 lab tests and say they are fine, with another endocrinologist testing nearly every bodily hormone including having patients collect urine for 24 hours to look for subtle changes in the production of adrenal hormones. It is also, often, the least necessary referral since many PCPs pride themselves on their knowledge of endocrinology. However, when fatigue is a major symptom, the endocrine system must be considered.

The major hormones that affect energy level come from the brain, a few glands in the neck and chest, the pancreas, and the adrenal glands. The difficult thing about testing these is that most hormones fluctuate dramatically in the course of a day, and the range of normal for many of them is hotly debated. The most common hormone problems that play a role in energy level are the thyroid hormone and the hormones in the pancreas that modify blood sugar (insulin in particular). These are the quickest and easiest to test, and primary care doctors will often test them in otherwise healthy individuals at yearly visits. However, when it comes to the steroids and other hormones made in the brain and adrenal glands, the first round of simple testing is often insufficient. Luckily, disorders related to cortisol, aldosterone, and sex hormones typically will have other severe body symptoms like changes to weight, skin color, and fat deposition that can be seen when a patient walks in the door.

Fundamentally, I have found that primary care doctors are typically great at identifying the most common endocrine disorders, and usually quite good at referring to endocrinology whenever there is a real question about some of the more rare conditions related to the pituitary gland or the adrenal glands. However, it is difficult for patients to know if they have had the right tests because of the complexity of those diagnoses, so having a clear and honest discussion about this with the PCP or an endocrinologist is often helpful. Asking "have we ruled out" Addisons, Cushings, Hypoaldosteronism, Diabetes Insipidus, Hyperprolactinemia, or Low-testosterone should be a very quick and simple discussion with the PCP, and I find trusting them when they say "those are unlikely" is typically sufficient.

Rheumatology

Some of the most important syndromes related to Long COVID symptoms, and many of the most important investigations into treatable components of the disorder, are in the field of rheumatology. Rheumatology has evolved dramatically, transitioning from a field of study related to swelling or "the flow of fluids" within joints and tissues (from which it derives its name) to a field primarily focused on inflammation throughout the body. For unclear reasons, they are often resistant to testing for or managing certain inflammatory conditions, especially in the brain (deferring to neurology), the stomach and intestines (deferring to gastroenterology), and in the skin or mucous membranes (which they defer to allergists or dermatologists). They also share many disorders with other disciplines like muscle inflammation (shared with neurology), joint pain (shared with orthopedics and anesthesiologists), and certain inflammatory disorders like sarcoidosis (shared with pulmonology). This can make identifying their role very difficult, but they are often helpful at making sure the inflammatory pattern does not fit a disorder for which there is a good immune system treatment.

One of the most difficult components of working with rheumatologic diagnoses is that many of them rely upon difficult to interpret blood tests. For example, a test called anti-nuclear antibodies (or ANA) is often run by PCPs and can be positive in many patients without primary rheumatologic disorders. Every few years, the criteria for rheumatologic conditions change based on new evidence in research, meaning that a primary care doctor or a neurologist may want to run a test that is deemed by the rheumatologist to be irrelevant. While they may, one day, take the reins in the management of Long COVID since it is considered to be caused by a misbehaving immune system, currently they are mainly helpful in ruling out other primary rheumatologic conditions such as lupus, rheumatoid arthritis, and many others.

When visiting with a rheumatologist, I find it is best for patients to have identified a few specific components of their Long COVID syndrome and to let the rheumatologist guide the discussion. Any body part (especially muscle or joint) that aches, swells, gets warm/cold, or turns red can be important to discuss with a rheumatologist since it can be a sign of inflammation. Also, any symptom that slowly escalates over a week, stabilizes for a month or so, and gradually improves may be very relevant since that is the typical time course for an "inflammatory event". Rashes or sores are important to identify, and taking very clear pictures of them is important because they might resolve by the time of the appointment. Dry mouth and eyes not caused by medications or seasonal changes are important to mention. Lastly, mention any symptoms that feel like an infection (called B-symptoms) such as night sweats, fevers, whole body aching, or shivering.

Rheumatology is unique in that they will often take a primary role in the management of disorders that are not truly rheumatologic in nature. Some act as chronic pain specialists, even when the cause of the symptoms are related to orthopedic injuries or from the brain, with fibromyalgia being the typical diagnosis given. They are also some of the best physicians to manage, monitor, and taper chronic steroid prescriptions regardless of why the steroids were started in the first place. They are particularly insightful when it comes to certain infections like Lyme disease, sometimes being more up to date in the literature than infectious disease doctors. However, at the end of the day their main role is to diagnose and treat any possible "primary rheumatologic conditions" that may be participating in the Long COVID syndrome.

Neurology

Neurology consults play a very peculiar role because the focus and training of any individual neurologist is extremely variable. The field of neurology began as a "broadening" of the training given to internal medicine doctors, but about 50 years ago neurologists began training less and less in general medicine and becoming more and more specialized. It started out as an "am I missing anything" referral from other doctors because neurologists were just as good at looking for cardiac causes of fainting as seizure. They were just as well trained in nearly all of the above systems as an internist. After a PCP had exhausted their knowledge, a neurologist was a sufficient referral to cover all bases. It used to be said that a neurologist was simply an internist who walked their patients, meaning they could find complex medical syndromes by how they affected global routine physical activities. The world of training in neurology is now different. Many go in knowing they want to specialize in seizure disorders and they even neglect training in general neurology. No longer is the question, "What caused the loss of consciousness?" but simply "Was it a seizure?"

This may seem overly critical, and there are plenty of good general neurologists out there that maintain their skills in endocrinology and cardiology, but it is the exception rather than the rule. Because of this, the neurology consultation should be considered very similar to the cardiology consult. Are there any neurologic conditions that should be ruled out, and can the neurologist help with any of the major neurologic components of the Long COVID syndrome? Keep in mind, with the split between neurology and psychiatry, the neurologist is not in charge of a majority of symptoms related to the brain, just the ones deemed to be primary neurologic syndromes. These include large and small fiber neuropathy or central neuropathic pain, certain types of cognitive decline (like Alzheimer's, strokes, etc...), primary vertigos, migraine and other atypical headaches, seizures, inflammation of the brain and spinal cord like multiple sclerosis or encephalitis, and some disorders of the muscle or the connection between the nerves and the muscles. Nearly all neurologists can "rule these out" quickly and easily, and most will be able to find the appropriate treatment for them.

The best way to prepare for the neurology visit is to organize your symptoms into groups by how they fluctuate over time. Do any symptoms come on suddenly and only last for a minute or two? Which symptoms escalate and resolve over the course of a few hours or weeks? Which symptoms are slowly progressive or constant? Try to consider how they could be related to the nervous system (brain, spinal cord, nerves), and if they do not seem to be, consider them as important but secondary symptoms. Heart symptoms, for example, can technically be related to the electrical system of the heart, but many neurologists would deem these "non-neurological". The same is true with primary psychiatric syndromes being a brain problem, and muscle (orthopedic) or inflammatory (rheumatologic) pain syndromes. All of these involve the nervous system, but most neurologists will dismiss them as non-neurologic conditions.

The most common syndrome a neurologist can help treat is migraine or atypical headache, but beyond that they have specific tools unique to the neurologist that can help diagnose or "rule out" important conditions. For questions of genuine cognitive decline, a neurologist may order formal "neuropsychological" testing to see if it fits a pattern such as Alzheimer's. MRIs are terrible at identifying the cause of brain fog or dementia, but they are great at looking for strokes or inflammation. PCPs will often order a brain MRI for headache or cognitive decline, but it is better for this test to be ordered by a neurologist because they will often ask for particular scans to be run for particular symptoms and they are able to look at the actual brain MRI and say if the radiologist report was accurate or relevant. However, if the physical neurologic exam is normal and the history is not consistent with strokes or tumors, MRIs can harm patients by finding common and non-dangerous "abnormalities" (incidentalomas) that lead to a lot of anxiety at best, and at worst more invasive testing like brain biopsies. EMG is the best test to identify any large nerve damage and some muscle disorders, and this is often followed by a small skin biopsy to look for any damage to the nerves in the skin. Lastly, any spells that could be seizure require an EEG and an interpreting neurologist, but like heart rhythm disorders, if the symptom is not occurring during the EEG, then the EEG may not be abnormal. All neurologists should be capable of identifying when and how to utilize neuropsychological testing, MRI, EMG, EEG, and lumbar puncture to look for treatable "primary neurological components" of the Long COVID syndrome.

I truly want to emphasize that while they are all well-trained and very smart, neurologists are very different regarding what their academic and intellectual focus is. All neurologists should be able to rule out seizure, multiple sclerosis, and small fiber neuropathy, but you may find a neurologist who truly is "an internist who walks his patients". However, just because they are really good at making the right diagnosis for a hormone disorder or a mood disorder does not mean they are capable of treating it as well as an endocrinologist or a psychiatrist. This mismatch between the neurologist's skill at identifying a problem and their ability to treat it has led to the criticism that they "diagnose and adios". This puts a great burden on the patient to carry this information back to the PCP, and a lot of pressure on the PCP, who may disagree with the diagnosis. It is truly better in most cases for the physician who runs the test to be the same one who can give the treatment.

Psychiatry

The reality, whether they like it or not, is that psychiatrists are the most experienced physicians regarding the safe and effective use of most of the medications used to treat Long COVID symptoms. They are more familiar with the escalation of medications like venlafaxine, the pharmaceutical treatment of insomnia, and monitoring mood changes and other side effects of dopamine-blocking and sodium-channel-modulating agents described in the medications chapter. Likewise, they are all trained to slowly deescalate medications that can be either harmful in Long COVID (like high dose chronic benzodiazepine or opiate therapies) or need to be stopped as they might interact with better medications (like switching from an SSRI to an SNRI). They are also used to routine coordination with therapists to monitor and enhance habit changes with exercise, meditation, sleep hygiene, and others. However, psychiatry has never played a major role in investigating or treating post-infectious chronic fatigue and pain syndromes. This, along with a psychiatrist shortage, poor incentivization for them to take insurance, and a preference to take care of only primary psychiatric patients makes finding a good psychiatrist who will treat Long COVID very difficult.

The discussion should begin with a psychotherapist as soon as a PCP feels they do not know the next steps to adjust treatment. Psychotherapists are often familiar with the local landscape of psychiatric prescribers, who are attentive to complex patients, and who seem to think in a complex way about unique patient situations. Often therapists also have a good referral system in place, so that patients do not end up on a 6 month waitlist. They know how to get patients other resources, like intensive outpatient programs. If a psychotherapist is willing to coordinate with a psychiatrist on treatment of Long COVID fatigue, insomnia, and depression symptoms, a patient has the best chance for recovery. In truth, psychiatry should have never split from neurology, and most neurologists would find that coordinating with psychotherapists could revolutionize the care of their patients.

Like with all providers, common factors are essential. The psychiatrist must understand the patient's goal and situation through thoughtful listening, must be compassionate, and must have the ability to negotiate a shared goal and treatment plan to achieve that goal. If the psychiatrist feels that Long COVID is too foreign to them, they can still help by identifying any psychiatric components and treating them as they would for any other patient. Even if the depression syndrome is mostly due to Long COVID, a psychiatrist treating depression independently can be quite helpful.

Beyond The Specialty Consultations

Most of the data surrounding effective treatment of post-infectious chronic fatigue syndromes suggests no one person can effectively treat it and the team approach is ideal. I began with specialty consultations because many patients and primary care doctors are worried that "something else is going on" and if there is another chronic condition that should be treated, identifying it and treating it is vital for recovery. However, most people simply have Long COVID, and waiting to receive treatment until you have spent a year going to specialists is counterproductive.

From the beginning, you should consider that you are building a team of providers. I will re-emphasize that this team should center around primary care, should include a practitioner of at least one physical treatment (personal trainer, massage therapist, chiropractor, and/or standard physical therapist to name a few), one psychotherapist, possibly a care coordinator or case manager, and a psychiatrist if the PCP's first few medication choices are not particularly helpful. This core team should be established within a month or two of the Long COVID diagnosis. If one team member is not fully effective, you should continue to work with the others while you look for a replacement.

Hopefully, by this point, you have identified your personal problem cycle. A common example is that migraine worsens fatigue, fatigue worsens insomnia, insomnia worsens migraine. Another is that fatigue makes someone sedentary, reduced activity increases snacking on unhealthy foods, and unhealthy foods worsen fatigue. A common resistance to treatment is referred to as the "yes, but" loop. "Yes, I should eat healthier, but I'm too tired to cook and nothing on Grubhub is healthy". "Yes I should exercise, but going outside makes my migraine worse." This is usually due to a symptom cycle that must be treated slowly by addressing all components simultaneously. Psychotherapists are particularly good at helping patients identify hurdles and come up with a plan to tackle them.

With this assembled team, especially if they can be coordinated, nearly all symptoms of Long COVID can be addressed. There will be plenty of trial and error, maybe switching team members if they are on a different page or cannot coordinate, or switching medications due to side effects. However, as long as everyone keeps working together, with shared goals, patients inevitably get better.

For most of my patients, scheduling regular appointments with each core team member is vital until symptoms have sufficiently improved. Patients should see the primary care team every 3 months to discuss any new symptoms or to re-evaluate specialty referrals, the psychiatrist once per month to adjust medications, the psychotherapist once per week to focus on skills and address barriers to habit changes, and a physical therapist or other physical practitioner once or twice per week to make sure they are staying active and not exhausting themselves. These can be more or less frequent depending on the focus of treatment, but research has shown a more comprehensive team approach is far more effective than just relying on one or two providers to monitor and guide every aspect.

Unfortunately, this ideal and comprehensive approach is rare. A few "Long COVID clinics" have popped up in every major city, but they will rarely have all of the different components of care centrally. They will often review every aspect and have one or two therapeutic interventions that they guide, and then they will direct patients to get a therapist, a physical therapist, and see a handful of specialists. They rarely have a psychiatrist in the group, and they may only have familiarity with one or two of the drugs used in the disorder. My experience with co-managing patients with "Long COVID clinics" is mixed, often with patients confused about who is doing and monitoring what. In truth, the current medical model is poorly designed to care for patients with complex multi-system syndromes requiring a lot of behavioral management and physical treatment.

CHAPTER 10: POTHOLES ON THE JOURNEY

If you have made it this far, you have hopefully learned that the science has progressed to give a good, however incomplete, picture of the cause of Long COVID and that millions are suffering just like you. There are many options for treatment, even when all the tests are coming back normal. Medications, physical therapies, psychotherapies, and other therapeutics can all help. While there are a dozen specialists that may or may not need to get involved briefly to rule out other medical conditions, most of the work can center around the primary care team, a psychotherapist, one or more physical therapists, and a psychiatrist if your PCP is uncomfortable with certain medications. The key to getting better is to assemble a team that will work together to monitor progress and adjust treatment as the disorder evolves. Easy peasy, right?

Of course not. If it were that simple, there would

not need to be a book to guide patients through the Long COVID journey. Before I discuss the problems in our medical system, I must be very clear about something. Nearly every medical provider I have met truly sees their work as a passion, wanting to do everything they can for their patients. They try to learn how to be compassionate caregivers, they have strong work ethics, and they would never do anything to break their vow to do no harm. Any deficits they have are due to how they are recruited, trained, and incentivized, and I do not believe it is their fault. Like with all large organizations, each person can be compassionate, and yet the system can be destructive. Unfortunately, it does not matter how compassionate any one cog is.

As I have said before, our medical system thrives if a patient's problem is only in one system. You have a liver problem, we have a liver doc. You have a heart problem, we have a heart doc on call for you. Unfortunately Long COVID is a whole body problem, and while PCPs are doing their best, there are not enough hours in the day for them to even do proper yearly physicals on all the patients under their care. A recent study showed that for the average primary care doctor to just do simple screenings based on the current guidelines, for the number of patients that the primary care doctors are typically responsible for, they would have to work 7 days a week for 26 hours per day. They must be the center of care for Long COVID, but they are in short supply. We were in a physician shortage before the pandemic. Now, due to burnout and an aging population of physicians some surveys have shown that close to 20% of primary care physicians plan to retire within the year. Long COVID may be a total system failure of the body, but it has also cast light onto the total system failure of our medical system.

The Long Covid Patient Experience

We know Long COVID is a very real disease with very real biological changes to the body and brain. Yet, so many patients leave the doctor's office feeling like they have been told nothing is wrong with them. This is not a criticism of those physicians, and it is definitely not a criticism of our patients. The physician runs the tests they know to run, or the ones they think will change management, and the tests come back normal. The patient hears that message as "nothing is wrong" with them. It is quite reasonable for patients to respond to this frustrating situation with anger and despair.

The infectious disease doctor has ruled out continued infection, even though the astrocytes are prone to direct infection, and this cannot be tested without biopsy. The pulmonologist has ruled out any treatable lung damage, even if some complex testing might show poor oxygen exchange. The cardiologist and the vascular specialists have ruled out any treatable and dangerous cardiac or vascular conditions, even though biopsies on patients show long-term effects from COVID-19 on all of those systems. The rheumatologist has ruled out any autoimmune syndrome (that they know how to treat), even though we know the immune system plays an important role in all of the symptoms of Long COVID. The sleep specialist has ruled out sleep apnea or narcolepsy, though the patient's sleep quality is terrible. Likewise, the neurologist could know everything about the neuroscience of COVID in the brain, but they have no way to treat activated microglia. Psychiatrists may know nothing about activated microglia, but they and the therapists they work with have the tools to treat the patient.

Unfortunately, post-infectious neurocognitive syndromes are not in the psychiatry manuals, and many psychiatrists rightfully feel unprepared to treat a "neurological condition". However, I have seen some of the worst disasters in medicine caused by non-psychiatrists trying to do their best to treat patients with psychiatric medications. Not only are the medications complex, but the possible interactions and side effects can even be life-threatening. Your physician might be aware of the Libby Zion case, especially if they have trained within the past 20 years. Modern medical residents are supposed to have an 80 hour limit on their work week because of one patient who died due to a resident's poor understanding (during a state of exhaustion) of the toxic effects of serotonin-modulating and dopamine-blocking medications. If care was better coordinated, and psychiatrists worked more closely with other specialists, those errors would not happen as often. However, our specialist driven system, with overwhelmed and burnt out primary care physicians, makes a coordinated treatment of Long COVID very difficult.

Reforms

I may sound like an idealist or a futurist, but I have become quite skeptical that we will overcome the problems in medicine with gradual change or routine scientific advancement. To paraphrase Einstein, you cannot solve a problem with the same kind of thinking used when creating the problem. A more accurate, however cynical, maxim from the famous physicist Max Planck goes as follows: "A new scientific truth does not triumph by convincing its opponents and making them see the light, but rather because its opponents eventually die, and a new generation grows up that is familiar with it." In our society, hospitals and insurance companies can never die to allow for new ideas to flourish. It is only at this higher institutional level that change could be made to globally impact a condition as common as Long COVID, and they seem to have no interest in pragmatism or efficiency.

One major problem is how physicians are trained and incentivized. Any practicing physician will joke about how little the medical school textbook prepares students for the practice of medicine. In practice, physicians are either paid by volume of work done, or one of many models designed to compensate them for their time or the value of their work, but all of these models have flaws. None of the payment models incentivize compassion, time spent helping patients understand their health, or helping complex patients change their habits to prevent illness. While preventing illness is much cheaper than treating it, our sick care industry has not found a way to adapt to it.

American healthcare is great for those wealthy enough to have a concierge primary care, pay out of pocket for Ph.D. level psychologists and physical therapists, and can hire lifestyle coaches, personal chefs, and personal trainers. For those unlucky enough to be born within the middle and working class, medicine is an assembly line with many broken conveyor belts. These assembly lines are inefficient at best, and too often directly harmful. If we cannot afford to train more physicians, therapists, and other medical providers and improve the machinery of medicine, then the whole system needs to be recreated from scratch. We definitely cannot afford the coming wave of baby boomer chronic illness, or the waves of novel and chronic infections and worsening psychiatric illnesses plaguing younger generations.

Can Medicine Be Reinvented?

At the core, one problem we have is how we identify and diagnose a new syndrome. At least sufferers from Long COVID have been lucky in this. The Long COVID syndrome was identified and accepted as a disease almost immediately without argument. It was a simple reaction to the flood of patients feeling they were still sick, and arguing they do not exist would be futile. Previously, similar infections such as Lyme disease, often followed by residual symptoms, were treated with more skepticism. Now, though the acute infection has wide agreement on its existence, the chronic post-infectious sequelae long after eradication of the bacteria is still considered nonsense by most modern physicians.

A condition being real, and how we determine the criteria for it, is determined by committee and those committees are prone to error. Often an obsession with a theory will pervade medical training such as the idea that Alzheimer's is caused by amyloid plaques in the brain. Many better theories have been proposed. Many disasters have occurred when trying to treat Alzheimer's by removing those plaques. Now, many reports of false or misleading seminal research articles have been published. Nevertheless, the amyloid hypothesis continues to receive the majority of funding in research, and is still taught as the mechanism of the disease in all medical schools.

Many diagnoses in psychiatry have degenerated due to their attempts to simplify or categorize disorders.

In his memoir *Darkness Visible*, novelist William Styron summed up the diagnosis of "depression" as well as any I have heard:

"Melancholia... was usurped by a noun with bland tonality and lacking any magisteria presence, used indifferently to describe an economic decline or a rat in the ground...The Swiss-born psychiatrist Adolf Meyer had a tin ear for the finer rhythms of English and therefore was unaware of the semantic damage he had inflicted by offering "depression" as a descriptive noun for such a dreadful and raging disease. Nonetheless, for over seventy-five years the word has slithered innocuously through the language like a slug, leaving little trace of its intrinsic malevolence and preventing, by its very insipidity, a general awareness of the horrible intensity of the disease..."

Melancholia is simply "depression" now, as is neurasthenia, catatonia, certain forms of psychosis, apathy, and the dysthymic personality disorder. The rich variety of human experience with negative emotional valence has been distilled down like a bad vodka, losing any subtleties that might exist in guiding treatment. In stark contrast, whole disorders in psychiatry have been invented by pharmaceutical companies in an effort to sell more drugs. Irritable bowel syndrome, social phobia/social anxiety disorder, and premenstrual dysphoric disorder are good examples of disorders that were not discussed until they happened to flood the literature alongside newly patented drugs which happened to be created for them.

Similarly, potentially life-changing treatments may be ignored in the literature if they are no longer patented, and no one will fund research comparing an old drug with a new drug if there is any chance of a financial drawback for the owner of the new drug. A recent analysis of rheumatoid arthritis patients showed that taking hydroxychloroquine had a 10-15% reduction in the development of Alzheimer's disease compared to other therapies, but there will never be a study comparing hydroxychloroquine to the new, controversial, expensive, and often dangerous infusion drugs. Along similar lines, in the early 2000s there was universal acceptance that melatonin is helpful for insomnia. Consequently, drugs that act by a similar mechanism like ramelteon were created and patented. However, no large trial comparing ramelteon and melatonin was ever performed, though melatonin's cost is $5 for 120 tabs and ramelteon's cost is $140 for 30 tabs.

From academia's incentives to focus on outdated theories to industry-guided diagnostic and treatment paradigms, the science of medicine has been fraught with bias. Unfortunately, all new theoretical models that diverge from this will fail, since the funding comes from the establishment. Some propose that incremental change can eventually override this, and others say we simply need fresh ideas. However, the financial medical-industrial complex will always resist any true reforms.

Redefining A Diagnosis

While it may seem absurd, there is a way around this. Let medicine continue to do what it is doing, but create a new research model. Machine learning is a novel analytic technique that can, if properly designed, reconceptualize human disease and treatment from a new unbiased perspective. If patients simply provided data about their symptoms, lifestyle, and medications, algorithms could identify patterns and phenomena in human health which could never be imagined in the ivory tower of academia. What if sadness is not a good way to predict a response to one antidepressant over another. Perhaps a "depression" with slowing of thought and movement changes responds better to certain medications while "depression" with irritability responds better to others. Some of these subtleties are considered by some psychiatrists, but neither medical research nor guideline considerations tackle these questions.

Through these machine learning algorithms, speech patterns have shown to better differentiate very early Parkinson's from other degenerative conditions. Who knows what a novel, unbiased reinvention of the medical scientific method would discover about the risks and disorders associated with aging and illness? Maybe it would perfectly mirror our current understanding of human physiology, but perhaps it would be more similar to Traditional Chinese Medicine, or completely alien to our current model of thought. This method would also quickly identify new infections before they become a pandemic, and would identify risks, trends, and patterns of new post-infectious syndromes associated with them.

Analyses of large populations already occur in other countries, though we are averse to them in freedom-loving America. For some reason, people are less bothered by Facebook and Google monitoring everything they say and do than they are by a governmental agency monitoring health. However, even Denmark population studies require a biased observer to determine which variables to consider. If this method were effective for identifying syndromes and treatments, we would not need to discard standard allopathic medicine, or even let the new medical science guide any treatments until the data supported a shift. However, unless we try we will never know if there is a better way.

Training And Incentivization In Medicine.

Likely the most frustrating barrier to innovation in medicine is the current model for recruiting and training physicians and researchers. To understand this, one must consider the path to becoming a physician with a critical, and perhaps cynical, eye. Again, I must emphasize that most of the people in the system are trying their best.

What are the qualities of the individuals accepted into medical school? There are only three that seem to matter based on reports of acceptance rates. Trainees in medicine must be very skilled at absorbing vast amounts of information through rote memory techniques, and regurgitating them on multiple choice tests. They must be very obedient, able to jump through every hoop thrown at them without complaint: building their CV, joining the right organizations, joining a research project, playing an instrument or having some sort of attractive hobby, etc. In addition, trainees must be able to charm at least three instructors who will write them recommendation letters. It also helps if they have a wealthy parent so they are not forced into indentured servitude to pay back the average of greater than $200,000 of student loans required to obtain the degree.

This system creates young physicians-in-training who are obedient, or at least able to hide disruptive thoughts. They toe the party line with regards to what they are taught, filling in the little circle for C when that was taught as the right answer, even if they believe it is wrong or do not understand it. Innovative thinking is pretty unhelpful in this. Having a mentor to help guide the process is vital, so the old guard shows the clear path. Money to pay for extra test-prep courses can mean the difference between acceptance and rejection. This is the way it has been done for the last 100 years since the current training model was invented by the leaders at John Hopkins after the disarray described in the Flexner report.

Of course, the ladder continues indefinitely for many of the brightest in academia, where falling in line is the best way to succeed. For others, jumping off the ladder means being a workhorse for a private hospital or medical group. In the past, physicians having their own private practices was routine, but now the majority of physicians rely upon the infrastructure of corporate entities to reduce the burden of running a business. There is a lot of manual labor associated with the billing sheet factory the modern medical industry has become.

Like all industries, medicine has a problem with their model of recruitment, training, and incentivization. Despite this, I have found most physicians to be generally very compassionate, hard working, and focused on the best interest of their patients. However, they are burning out because of a system that abuses them, forces them to spend more time making billing sheets than making patients healthy, and penalizes innovation. There is no quick answer to this, and it likely will not come from within the medical establishment. It also cannot come from an industry that relies upon third-party payers only interested in quarterly profits, or a government run by lawyers and lobbyists. Interval improvement by making medical education free, less reliant upon hoop jumping, and less reliant upon the militaristic hierarchy that created our current model would at least help us rely upon the Planck model of scientific advancement.

Care Coordination And Integration

Without integrated care and coordination between providers (specialists, psychologists, physical therapists, and others), we will never be able to help those suffering from Long COVID. The two main barriers with regards to chronic illness management, neither of which are emphasized in medical training, are poor application of the allostatic load model of chronic disease and behavior modification training such as motivational interviewing. Many medical students and recent graduates will immediately balk at the latter part of that statement, since they had to learn the 4 processes (engaging, focusing, evoking, and planning), the 5 principles (empathy, discrepancy, resistance, self-efficacy, and autonomy), and the 6 stages (precontemplative, contemplative, preparation, action, maintenance, and termination) of motivational interviewing. They aced that portion of the multiple choice practice tests. These young doctors are unaware of another classical concept, and I urge them to learn about the Dunning-Kruger effect.

In the meantime, I will happily die on this hill. Medical trainees are taught they must understand every chemical in the mitochondria that turns sugar into energy, but they are only given the most cursory instruction of how to help patients address unhealthy habits. As we have discussed, diet, exercise, sleep, and other habits are likely the most important and most neglected components of health and well-being, and clearly learning the answers to 15 possible multiple choice questions has not done the trick. There was a burst of interest in changing the language physicians use, such as eliminating the term non-compliance in favor of non-adherence. Surprisingly, this was also insufficient to transform masters of the multiple choice question into good behavioral analysts or even psych 101 level behaviorists.

Changing Habits

Motivational interviewing is an overly distilled simplification of philosophical concepts present throughout the fields of psychology. In its essence, it is an acceptance that intellect and character are brain functions that are somewhat distinct from behavioral programming. Discussed in philosophy since before the ancient Greeks, many will recognize early religious examples: "For what I do is not the good I want to do; no, the evil I do not want to do - this I keep on doing." While Paul and others attribute this to some ephemeral sinfulness or karma, our modern understanding is simply related to brain circuits for reward and behavioral habit sequencing.

Unfortunately, we do not have a scalpel small enough to modify those circuits yet. Luckily, the various fields of human and animal psychology have formulated a hundred different models of addressing these issues. None of it is truly taught to young doctors.

A better education in the practical applications of human psychology might be the only way to resolve this deficit. I have met some physicians who developed their own framework for understanding human behavior and motivation, often after their lives were decimated by addiction. However, expecting physicians to only have an awareness of holes they have already fallen into strikes me as foolish.

This education would have to start at the earliest stages, possibly as early as high school when most people formalize their concept of what makes people "do what they do". This is the height of when they break from their parent's perception of who is good and bad, and formulate their own opinions, if they do at all. During this developmental stage, they could ideally shed their biases against obesity (likely more related to the gut microbiome than lack of willpower), personality disorders (a normal biological response to trauma which gives an evolutionary advantage to the species), volition (the retrospective justification of innate and unconscious drive reduction), and other common misperceptions related to human behavior. At least it would give them a better understanding of what does and does not motivate behavioral change.

I had to spend 12 months learning physics, ostensibly to understand how an MRI machine works. It would be far more practical to spend 12 months exploring the science of how people work.

The Allostatic Load

The second neglected concept, required to understand the problems with coordinated care, is the theory of allostatic load. Since the Framingham study began in the late 1940s, the principles of allostatic load have been taught cursorily to young physicians. However, they are not really educated on its implications throughout the rest of medicine. In short, 5000 residents of the town Framingham, Massachusetts were recruited to monitor a variety of risk factors related to heart health. It had been determined that blood pressure, blood sugar, lack of exercise, and smoking all increased the risk of heart disease, but no one really knew which were the most important. When the data showed they are all roughly equal, but compounded in a greater way than addition alone, a theory had to be developed to explain this. In Western medicine, we want so badly to separate things, but the living human body is one interconnected, integrated system that cannot be easily divided into parts. While we can see parts of these systems working together, the true symphony of the human body is too complex to understand outside of broad metaphors, and the best metaphor for these interactions and their effects on various medical conditions is the allostatic load model.

Why does depression increase the risk of stroke? Why does childhood trauma increase the risk of diabetes? Why does access to fruits and vegetables (not just eating them) reduce the risk of cancer? The Western allopathic model of medicine would want a clear and linear answer based on our knowledge of human biology. Maybe depression increases cortisol, resulting in free radicals, which damage the lining of the blood vessel walls, which leads to plaque formation, resulting in stroke. However, that is all made-up, post-hoc determinism, lazy reasoning at best, a teleological fallacy at worst. The reality is we do not understand how it works.

Enter the allostatic load model of human health. Imagine a dozen or more mechanisms that individually balance the body's primary functions. Temperature, blood pressure, blood sugar, mood regulation, adaptive responses to trauma each a balancing act. When blood sugar rises a bit too high, insulin is secreted by the pancreas to lower it. If it dips too low, glucagon is secreted to raise it. This balancing act of the body is called a homeostatic mechanism. Each homeostatic mechanism is taught as an independent circuit in the body. In the allostatic load model of human health, one of the balancing mechanisms can falter and there are few down-stream effects. If you disrupt two or three, then the other circuits begin to falter. Disrupt four or five and the whole system begins to fail. The Framingham study described this perfectly for heart disease, but similar analyses have supported this model with regards to everything from cancer risk to the manifestation of genetic disorders.

An Argument For Integrated Care

What does all this have to do with coordination of care? Simply speaking, if I am responsible to care about a patient's diabetes risk, then I must care about their psychological health, their physical activity, their diet, and all other systems that may have a connection to it. When I prescribe a blood sugar medication, I test the patient's blood sugar a month later, tracking and honing my approach until the right dose is found and the patient says they tolerate any side effects. For some reason, the same vigilance is rarely applied to a recommendation that a patient receive physical therapy, psychotherapy, or nutritional counseling. Typically, the best physicians do is see if the patient even saw the therapist. An amazing physician may ask if the patient likes the therapist. Rarely does a physician ask what is happening in the therapy sessions, or monitor the results.

In the same way a medical student learns the different mechanisms of metformin, insulin, sitagliptin, and semaglutide, they should learn the different mechanisms of CBT, psychodynamic therapy, chiropractic treatments, and the utilization of kinesiology tape. Sure, as I have gotten further from medical school, I have to look up the mechanism of action and standard use of drugs like sitagliptin, but if I prescribed it as often as I recommend psychotherapy, I should know what it does, how it works, the risks and benefits of treatment, and other available options. Likewise, any physician who routinely recommends patients find a therapist (physical therapy or psychotherapy) should have a cursory understanding of those disciplines.

If physician education emphasized the psychology of behavior modification and the importance of integrated systems, doctors would be fully aware of why Americans die of heart disease at rates greater than any other in the world despite having the "best medical care in the world". The logic is inescapable.

Access To Care

I have interviewed many patients about their experiences struggling to navigate the complex medical system. Books could be written on each state's policies regarding medicare, medicaid, and private insurance with regards to what is covered, how it is covered, and potential gaps in coverage. Unfortunately, if the books take more than a month to publish, this moving target would make them irrelevant. There is also an inordinate amount of misinformation and misunderstanding about what patients do and do not have access to, typically until it is too late.

Now, I do not want to be too political in this book about healthcare, but at its core, this is a political issue. One side of the aisle hopes for a single-payer healthcare system but has given no indication of how it would be run better than our broken multi-payer system. The other side offers internally inconsistent nonsense, promising cheap care and delivering nothing. Neither offer an efficient model of providing healthcare, and neither would resolve the problems with the fee-for-service model or the hospital industrial complex. I reject both wholeheartedly, but I still vote against anyone wanting politicians to have authority over patients and doctors.

The reality is that we have about five problems, and fixing one would not address the others.

1. Fundamentally we have too few physicians and other providers, which creates a supply and demand issue, along with an ethical dilemma insisting physicians see as many patients as possible, and that they not complain that corporations shackle them.
2. We have too many people profiting off of a "sick care" system, where each branch of each insurance/pharmaceutical/hospital corporation takes a bite of the apple.
3. Payment models encourage many visits with few solutions, often delaying standard care

until it is too late.

4. Political and insurance company demands are constantly changing, designed to only put burdens on physicians and patients.

5. Cartels and monopolies are disguised as non-profit institutions, leading to giant systems that have little regard for what happens "in the room".

Alone Together

For my Long COVID patients, all they see is neglect (or outright abuse) from the system, but they do not know why. Their COBRA insurance costs more than their disability check, but they do not qualify for Medicaid. None of their doctors seem to take Workers' Comp. They have not seen their PCP in a year because they do not have openings, and each time it is a different nurse practitioner. The disability insurance company wants the same form filled out again, and they worry their doctor is getting annoyed by all of the paperwork. For someone who does not have the energy to brush their teeth every day, all of these hurdles are truly insurmountable. Some patients give up and fall into institutionalization or become like a child to their spouse. Other patients push through, either as a lifeless automaton or bursting with rage at every person they interact with.

It does not have to be this way, but turning the labyrinth of the sick care system into an efficient health care system would take a more comprehensive overhaul than fixing any of the individual problems we have discussed. It must begin by addressing the core features of the workforce shortage, a look at who is profiting unduly from the sick care system, recognizing what can and should be automated, and developing systems of delivery that are effective and not simply profitable.

Public Health Innovations

The first problem is a simple mathematical equation. There are a certain number of patients, with a certain number of needs, and only a certain number of provider appointments to fill those needs. Under the current model, there is an increasing disparity between available care and needed care. Public health departments have long recognized this, and since they cannot arrange medical appointments for all of the population, they advertise on television. They create campaigns to end smoking, or reduce disease transmission.

However, while these measures do work, they clearly have not had enough of an effect. They are also poorly done. Our public health institutions have an almost comedic history with films like *Reefer Madness* or videos recorded in the '70s with teenagers talking about the dangers of sex and driving without a seatbelt. During the COVID pandemic, nearly everyone found issue with the Public Health response, which attempted to focus on simple messages like "flatten the curve" by wearing a cloth mask. Unfortunately, most of the information was incomplete or misleading causing more distrust from the population. However, since it would take decades to overhaul medical training to make a sufficient number of physicians, an automated approach is necessary.

It seems the only option is to learn from these mistakes and make an automated system of health advice and care delivery that learns and adapts over time. This could start in tandem with an automated data acquisition model, described earlier, for overhauling medical research. Patients enter their own medical history, family history, medications, and other pertinent details into a centralized database, and a recommended regimen could be automatically produced. This could be accompanied by personal biometric devices or mass clinics where certain measurements are taken such as blood pressure, weight, and simple blood tests done at yearly physicals.

This automated primary care system could have very few physicians involved, freeing them up to spend more time with complex or chronically ill individuals. Also, the rich history gained by the automated system would allow for them to spend more time getting to know the patient as an individual rather than filling out check lists in front of the patient. This would take time to implement, but with machine learning becoming advanced enough to predict which ads we will click on, the possibilities in automating routine health screenings are endless.

Before this can occur, public sentiment in politics must change. Our current system is wasteful and inefficient by design. Inefficiency in any system is a source of financial profit for many. If I could cure all diseases with a single pill, all other drug companies would go out of business. If an insurance company is able to keep 20% of their gross receipts as profit, they want the total cost of care to increase so their 20% slice increases. They can all pretend they want to improve the system, but if improving the system means lower profits, they will hire lobbyists to actively sabotage reform. This is a complex problem, but it can be made simple by initiating campaign finance reforms, making private lobbying illegal, and making any corporate healthcare companies compete with a new government run healthcare system that focuses on providing low cost automated care with high quality physician encounters.

Can We Automate Our Way Out?

So, consider Long COVID. Imagine a person is living their life, working at a good job, raising a family. A pandemic comes and they try to do everything right, but they are getting mixed messages from the news and their boss is making policies that put them at risk. Because they have high blood pressure and diabetes, they are at very high risk for more severe COVID-19 and developing the Long COVID syndrome. All they know is they cannot do their job anymore, webMD says they probably have brain cancer, and they just found out their PCP retired last year and someone will get back to them when they identify who can be their new PCP. The Urgent Care doctor ordered the same tests twice and they still came back normal. What now?

Now imagine during the early stages of the pandemic an automated system (called the "ePatient Advocate" or ePA) alerted the patient to the risks, what to expect, and some basic health measures they could do to prevent disease. It reminded them they had not gotten blood work in a few years and automatically identified their risk factors without needing to wait for a doctor's appointment (but a program established a PCP for the patient). The ePA began guiding the patient to an exercise routine and some basic ways to adjust diet to improve overall health. It automatically scheduled a virtual nurse practitioner visit starting safe medications for early diabetes and blood pressure. A ring on their finger (sent at the beginning of the pandemic) identified a fever early in the course of their infection and alerted their case manager to reach out to monitor symptoms. Paxlovid was quickly determined to be appropriate and it was prescribed.

Unfortunately, Long COVID still occurred even though they did everything right, but they were alerted to the symptoms by the ePA. That system sent a message to the case manager who helped schedule a PCP visit to get to know them and help clarify any information they did not understand from the ePA. The patient had already been scheduled for a physical therapy appointment because of muscle pain and fatigue, a psychotherapy appointment because of a positive depression screen, and a nutritionist appointment because the patient has not had any success trying to cook tasty and healthy foods. Because the heart rate jumps when the patient stands, a cardiology appointment was scheduled and a scan of the lungs was ordered to make sure there was no pneumonia or heart failure. Maybe all of these steps would have happened without the ePA, but the patient felt supported, the appointments happened quickly, and instead of three urgent care visits and an emergency department visit, all of the care was provided at home. Is it too expensive to provide automated care? Not as expensive as a single ED visit.

Changes We Can Make Now

Obviously this system would need to be developed very carefully, and there are many pit-falls. However, portions have already been shown to be effective. Programs like the Curable App have shown great success in managing chronic pain symptoms and educating patients about the nature of the disorder in simple language. Large insurance companies have created algorithms to identify medical risk, but they use it primarily to optimize profits and not to improve care. Other countries have worked on improving the automation of routine medical screenings, with or without medical doctors involved.

Many things cannot be automated. Basic education can, but answering follow-up questions cannot. However, even when something needs a personal touch, it can often be done with groups. Some of the best care I have seen in the current medical system occurs with Shared Medical Appointments (SMAs) where 10 or so patients participate in group visits, part group therapy, part support group, while one or more doctors, nutritionists, and physical therapists teach them together about diabetes care. While these providers do their care, the patients commiserate about their loss of chocolate cake and teach each other strategies for how to safely start a walking group in their neighborhood. In a SMA, you get an hour to an hour and a half per appointment, and the doctor can see 10 people in that time rather than 4-6. Similarly, chronic pain SMAs and multiple sclerosis SMAs have been validated as being more effective than quicker 15-minute individual follow-ups with the doctor.

The reality is that all of the pieces have been created, from AI and machine learning, automated education and advice, to models of group care. Physicians are already so overwhelmed by advances in medicine that most standards of care are automated through checklists, and many of these could be automated allowing for those doctors to spend more time engaging with patients on more unique struggles. Unfortunately, if this model were implemented in today's political climate, a dozen industrial groups would find ways to siphon off money and resources or create gold level automated care that only the rich can afford. It all seems impossible.

But it is not impossible if we remember our history. "We do these things not because they are easy, but because they are hard." Those were the words spoken by John F. Kennedy when he told the world that America could fly a man to the moon. This required a new government organization, innovative thinkers from many disciplines, coordination between private and public industries, and an understanding that the will of the American people could overcome resistance and negativity to create something undreamt of before. We did the same to build our postal system, our railway system, our bridges and tunnels, and even the atomic bomb. None of these could have developed if people were bound by the same level of thinking that created the problems that needed solving. There were definitely profiteers, but with good organizational leadership, with a singular goal, and with a mandate from the people, they were all achievable. Systemic restructuring in medical care is no less urgent than any of those, and is no less possible.

My hope with this chapter was not to simply shed light on the problems we face in medical care with training, structuring, and access, but to remind people what can be done when innovation is incentivised. Any individual living with Long COVID must now do for themselves what a system of care could do in the future. If we do not change, the whole system will become bankrupt and break apart like our bridges are doing now. However, with innovations in computing, automated guidance, and biometrics, we no longer need hope. All we need now is resolve.

Made in the USA
Las Vegas, NV
02 May 2024